Copernicus Books

Sparking Curiosity and Explaining the World

Drawing inspiration from their Renaissance namesake, Copernicus books revolve around scientific curiosity and discovery. Authored by experts from around the world, our books strive to break down barriers and make scientific knowledge more accessible to the public, tackling modern concepts and technologies in a nontechnical and engaging way. Copernicus books are always written with the lay reader in mind, offering introductory forays into different fields to show how the world of science is transforming our daily lives. From astronomy to medicine, business to biology, you will find herein an enriching collection of literature that answers your questions and inspires you to ask even more.

Guid Oei

The Artificial Womb

Life Saving for Extreme
Premature Babies

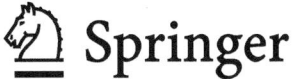 Springer

Guid Oei
Fundamental Perinatology
Máxima Medical Center,
University of Technology Eindhoven
Eindhoven, The Netherlands

ISSN 2731-8982   ISSN 2731-8990   (electronic)
Copernicus Books
ISBN 978-3-031-85904-5   ISBN 978-3-031-85905-2   (eBook)
https://doi.org/10.1007/978-3-031-85905-2

Cover illustration: *The "Recent Memory" for which the author, owner of the canvas, gives us permission* (Guid Oei, as the owner of the artwork entitled "Recent Memory," an oil on canvas by Mark Kostabi (2006), from my private collection, hereby grant my permission for the use of this artwork in the book entitled "The Promise of the Artificial Womb," authored by Guid Oei).
All other illustrations in this book are credited to Twan Oei.

This Springer imprint is published by the registered company Springer Nature Switzerland AG
The registered company address is: Gewerbestrasse 11, 6330 Cham, Switzerland

If disposing of this product, please recycle the paper.

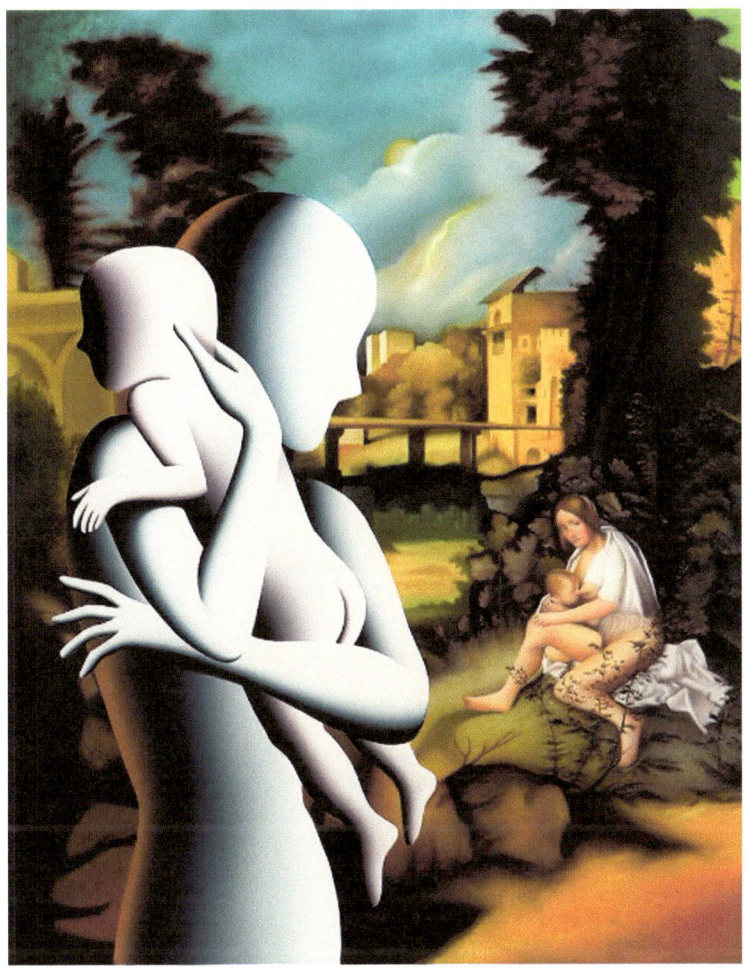

The cover features "Recent Memory," an oil on canvas by Mark Kostabi (2006), from a private collection.

For my patients

.

Preface

Over the past 30 years, as an obstetrician specializing in preterm birth, I have too often found myself powerless to prevent the tragedy of extremely preterm deliveries—many of which ended in heartbreaking loss. Despite decades of scientific progress, we remain unable to fully prevent preterm birth or mitigate its harmful consequences. Advances in neonatal care have undoubtedly improved survival rates, but far too many infants still face lifelong complications as a result of being born too soon.

This persistent sense of helplessness led me to search for new solutions beyond what conventional neonatal care could offer.

I began to explore how we might extend fetal development in an environment that closely mimics the womb—where a premature infant could continue growing as if birth had never occurred. This vision led to a collaboration between Máxima Medical Center, a hospital renowned for its expertise in preterm birth, and Eindhoven University of Technology, a leader in perinatal care innovation. By bringing together doctors and engineers, this partnership laid the foundation for extraordinary scientific advancements, ultimately aiming to develop a natural alternative to the incubator: an artificial womb that replicates the in utero environment to support preterm infants' growth and development.

Pivotal moments in this journey are the successful defenses of PhD dissertations at Eindhoven University of Technology, which delved into the interdisciplinary challenges and opportunities of developing perinatal life support systems. The research emphasized how design, integrated with co-creation, can drive transformative innovations. The project engaged a diverse range of stakeholders, including parents, obstetricians, neonatologists, engineers, and ethicists, to address the intricate challenges of creating an artificial womb.

This work highlighted an essential truth: solving a problem as complex as sustaining life outside the womb requires interdisciplinary collaboration. No single field can tackle this challenge alone. By involving end-users—parents and healthcare professionals—early in the development process, the research demonstrated that solutions could be both effective and more readily adopted in clinical practice.

The lessons learned from this collaboration serve as an example of how combining expertise, creativity, and co-creation can lead to meaningful progress in addressing some of the most complex issues in healthcare.

Around the world, only a handful of research groups are working on artificial placenta and womb technologies, each contributing unique expertise. If we hope to accelerate progress and bring these innovations to clinical practice, international collaboration is essential. By sharing resources, insights, and technologies, we can develop solutions that are accessible to all, particularly in low- and middle-income countries, where the burden of prematurity is highest.

This book focuses primarily on the development of artificial placenta and artificial womb technologies, which could address one of the most pressing global health issues: preterm birth, the leading cause of child mortality and long-term health complications worldwide. The "why" behind this research is undeniable. The urgent need to reduce neonatal mortality and morbidity compels us to innovate and act.

Although the book also briefly touches on the broader concept of complete ectogenesis—the idea of gestating a fetus entirely outside the body—it is important to clarify that no research group is currently pursuing this goal. While complete ectogenesis may one day be technically feasible, the "why" behind it is not yet compelling enough to justify significant investment. Without a clear and pressing problem to solve, such a pursuit remains speculative at best.

In contrast, the development of artificial placenta and womb technologies addresses a critical and immediate need. Preterm birth continues to be a leading cause of infant mortality and lifelong disability. The potential to reduce suffering and improve outcomes for these vulnerable infants is what drives researchers forward.

To make the subject accessible and engaging for a broad audience, this book is structured into ten chapters, each beginning with a fictional story based on real scientific possibilities. These stories serve as an imaginative lens through which readers can connect emotionally with the potential of artificial womb technology. Following each story, factual background information is provided, offering a detailed exploration of the scientific, ethical, and societal aspects of the topic. This dual approach aims to educate while sparking curiosity and reflection, ensuring that even complex scientific concepts are approachable for non-experts.

This book explores the intersection of science, ethics, and society in the quest to develop artificial womb technology. It celebrates the ingenuity of researchers while reflecting on the profound ethical questions raised by these innovations. By fostering international collaboration and co-creation, we can move closer to solutions that benefit everyone, regardless of geography or resources.

As you read this book, I encourage you to reflect on both the extraordinary possibilities and the immense responsibilities that come with these advancements. Innovation in perinatal care is not just a technological challenge; it is a moral one. Let us strive to ensure that the pursuit of progress is guided by empathy, respect, and a shared commitment to improving the lives of future generations.

Eindhoven, The Netherlands   Guid Oei

Acronyms, Abbreviations, and Key Terms

AAF —Artificial Amniotic Fluid A synthetic fluid designed to replicate the protective environment of natural amniotic fluid, supporting fetal development by regulating temperature and cushioning the fetus.

Alveoli Tiny, balloon-like structures in the lungs where the exchange of oxygen and carbon dioxide takes place. Alveoli are surrounded by a network of capillaries that transport blood, allowing oxygen to enter the bloodstream and carbon dioxide to be expelled from the body. In full-term infants and adults, alveoli are fully developed and number in the hundreds of millions, providing a large surface area for efficient gas exchange. However, in extremely preterm infants, the alveoli are not yet formed, and the lungs are in the canalicular stage of development, which limits their ability to support breathing and increases the risk of respiratory complications like Respiratory Distress Syndrome (RDS).

APAW —Artificial Placenta and Artificial Womb Combined systems designed to support fetal development by mimicking the functions of the natural placenta and uterus.

AP —Artificial Placenta A life-support system that oxygenates blood and removes waste, replacing the natural placenta's role in fetal development.

Apgar Score Named after Dr. Virginia Apgar, the Apgar score is a quick assessment tool used to evaluate a newborn's health immediately after birth. It measures five key criteria: skin color (appearance), heart rate (pulse), reflex irritability (response to stimuli), muscle tone (activity), and breathing effort (respiration). Each criterion is scored from 0 to 2, resulting in a total score ranging from 0 to 10. This score helps medical professionals determine whether a newborn needs urgent medical care. AW —Artificial Womb An environment that recreates the conditions of the uterus, providing a safe space for premature infants to grow.

CS —Caesarean Section A surgical method of childbirth involving an incision in the mother's abdomen and uterus, often used for complicated births.

ECMO —Extracorporeal Membrane Oxygenation A medical technique that uses a machine to take over the functions of the heart and lungs, providing oxygenation outside the body.

Ectogenesis The process of developing a fetus entirely or partially outside the natural womb, using an artificial environment to support growth and development. Ectogenesis holds potential for revolutionizing neonatal care, particularly for extremely preterm infants.

- **Complete Ectogenesis**:
  The concept of sustaining a fetus from conception to full term entirely outside the mother's body. This would involve replicating the entire gestational process in an artificial womb. Complete ectogenesis remains a theoretical possibility and is not yet being actively pursued due to significant technical, ethical, and societal challenges.

- **Partial Ectogenesis**:
  The process of supporting a fetus that has been partially gestated in the natural womb but requires continued development outside the body due to preterm birth. Partial ectogenesis aims to bridge the gap between extreme prematurity and full-term development, offering a more natural and less harmful alternative to current neonatal intensive care technologies. This approach is the primary focus of current research on artificial placenta and artificial womb systems.

ELGAN —Extremely Low Gestational Age Newborn A newborn born at less than 28 weeks of gestation. ELGANs are at high risk for severe complications due to their underdeveloped organs, including respiratory distress, brain hemorrhage, and infections. Specialized care, including advanced neonatal support systems, is crucial for their survival and long-term health.

GA —Gestational Age The age of the fetus measured in weeks from the first day of the mother's last menstrual period.

IVH —Intraventricular Hemorrhage A type of brain bleed occurring in premature infants, often originating from the fragile blood vessels in the germinal matrix—a highly vascularized area in the developing brain. IVH can lead to long-term neurological complications, with severity classified into four grades based on the extent of bleeding and ventricular involvement.

LFC —Liquid-Filled Chamber A controlled environment filled with artificial amniotic fluid where a fetus can develop in conditions similar to the womb.

LFL —Liquid-Filled Lungs A state where the lungs remain fluid-filled, as in the womb, to prevent injury and promote natural development during artificial gestation.

MV —Mechanical Ventilation The use of a machine to assist breathing in infants or patients with respiratory challenges.

NEC —Necrotizing Enterocolitis A severe gastrointestinal condition primarily affecting premature infants, in which portions of the intestine become inflamed, leading to tissue death. NEC can cause life-threatening complications, including infection and bowel perforation. Early diagnosis and treatment are critical to improve outcomes.

NICU —Neonatal Intensive Care Unit A specialized unit in hospitals designed to provide intensive medical care for premature and critically ill newborns.

NIDCAP —Newborn Individualized Development Care and Assessment Program A framework emphasizing customized care for newborns based on their individual developmental needs and family involvement.

PDA —Patent Ductus Arteriosus A condition in which the ductus arteriosus, a fetal blood vessel that bypasses the lungs, fails to close after birth. PDA is common in premature infants and can lead to complications such as heart failure and poor oxygenation, as it allows abnormal blood flow between the aorta and pulmonary artery. Treatment may include medication or surgery, depending on severity.

PMA —Postmenstrual Age

PLS —Perinatal Life Support An integrated system combining artificial placenta and artificial womb technology for extremely preterm infants.

RCT —Randomized Controlled Trial

RDS —Respiratory Distress Syndrome A common and serious condition in preterm infants caused by underdeveloped lungs that lack sufficient surfactant, a substance that prevents the alveoli in the lungs from collapsing. Without adequate surfactant, breathing becomes difficult, leading to oxygen deprivation. RDS primarily affects babies born before 34 weeks of gestation and is particularly severe in those born before 28 weeks. Treatments include surfactant replacement therapy and mechanical ventilation, though both can have long-term complications.

SEMS —Synthetic Embryo Models Laboratory-created structures that mimic key features of natural embryos during early development. Unlike natural embryos, SEMs are formed from stem cells without the use of eggs or sperm. These models are used to study early embryonic processes, organ formation, and developmental disorders, offering insights into reproduction and potential applications in regenerative medicine.

UC —Umbilical Cord The vital lifeline connecting the fetus to the placenta, delivering oxygen and nutrients while removing waste.

VB —Vaginal Birth Natural delivery of a baby through the birth canal.

Contents

1

The Perils of Extreme Prematurity: Understanding the Risks and the Need for Breakthrough Solutions

1.1 A Sudden Turn of Events

Anna and David had eagerly awaited this chapter of their lives—their first child was due in just a few months, and the future seemed full of promise. At 24 weeks into a smooth and uneventful pregnancy, they were savoring every moment of anticipation. To celebrate this milestone, they treated themselves to a quiet evening at their favorite restaurant, a ritual of small, meaningful celebrations during the pregnancy. But that evening would become etched in their memories for reasons they could never have imagined (Fig. 1.1).

As they lingered over their meal, laughter gave way to concern. Anna shifted uncomfortably in her chair and felt a sudden, unfamiliar warmth. At first, she dismissed it, assuming the chair was wet or that she had spilled water. But when she stood up, a trickle turned into a rush. Confusion quickly transformed into dread—could her water have broken? Alarmed, they stepped outside and called their midwife. Her response was firm but calm: they needed to go to the hospital immediately.

The drive to the hospital was tense and quiet. David's knuckles whitened on the steering wheel as he glanced nervously at Anna. The hospital staff moved swiftly, ushering them into an examination room. An internal examination confirmed their fears—amniotic fluid was leaking. Worse still, contractions had started, irregular but real.

The cardiotocogram (CTG), a monitor tracking the baby's heart rate, showed a strong heartbeat of 160 beats per minute. There were no signs of distress, no decelerations. Every 5–10 min, a contraction registered on the screen, and while they were not regular, they were enough to tighten Anna's jaw with discomfort. Further

© The Author(s), under exclusive license to Springer Nature Switzerland AG 2025
G. Oei, *The Artificial Womb*, Copernicus Books,
https://doi.org/10.1007/978-3-031-85905-2_1

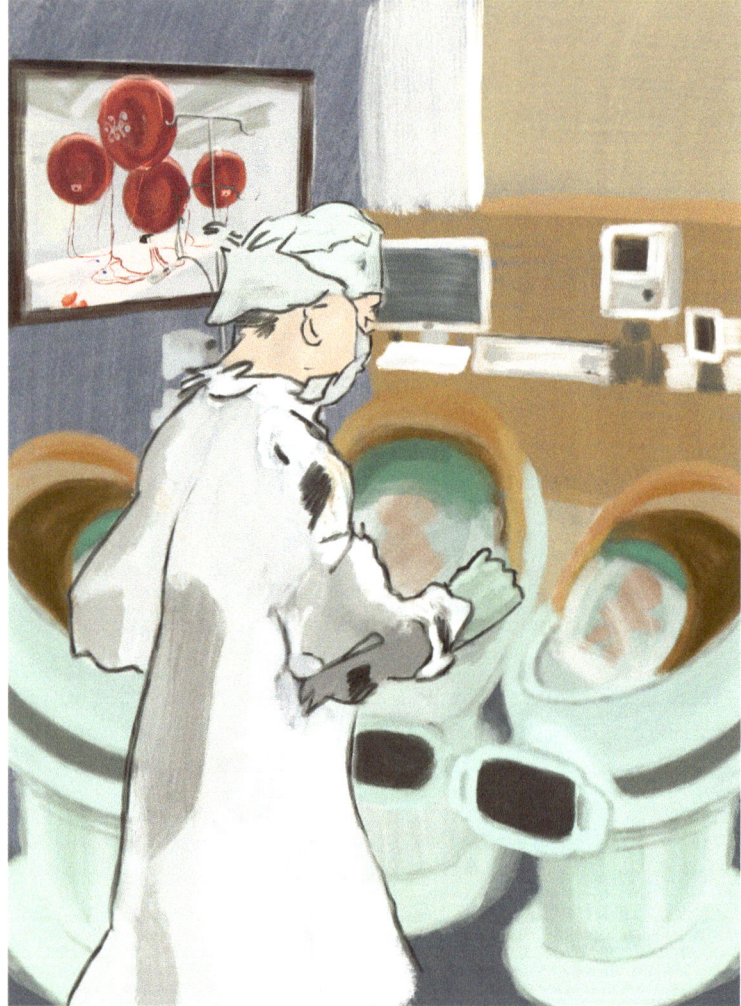

Fig. 1.1 Inside a fetal intensive care unit designed for artificial wombs, where innovative technologies and specialized medical teams work toward supporting the growth and development of extremely premature infants, underscoring the need for continued breakthroughs in neonatal care. The artificial womb design was created by Juliette van Haren, Assistant Professor at Eindhoven University of Technology

examination revealed 2 centimeters of cervical dilation. The room, filled with the beeping of monitors and hurried footsteps, seemed to close in around them.

Recognizing the critical situation, the obstetric team immediately contacted the regional perinatal referral center—Anna's pregnancy had become high-risk, and specialized care was essential. The answer came back quickly, and it was not what they hoped to hear: no beds were available. As Anna gripped David's hand, staff frantically searched for another option. Finally, after what felt like hours but was only minutes, a place was found—300 kilometers away. An ambulance was arranged, and Anna was prepared for the long journey.

David followed behind the ambulance, the kilometers stretching endlessly. Each one felt like a countdown, each moment an eternity of uncertainty. At the perinatal center, Anna was reassessed. Her dilation had progressed to 4 centimeters, and the contractions were stronger. Yet, the baby's heart continued to beat steadily, offering a fragile thread of hope.

An obstetrician and a neonatologist entered the room. Both had faces lined with the weight of difficult conversations and countless lives saved—and sometimes lost. They spoke with precision and compassion. "If your baby is born now, at 24 weeks," the perinatologists explained, "the survival rate is about 50%. But survival is only the beginning of the challenges. One in three babies born this early will have a severe disability, such as cerebral palsy or profound cognitive impairments. Another third may face mild disabilities, such as learning difficulties or motor challenges. And one in three may have no significant disabilities."

The words hung in the air, heavy and unavoidable. The doctors continued, explaining the options. "If you choose active intervention, we will do everything possible to give your baby a chance. This includes administering corticosteroids to speed lung development and tocolytics to delay labor. We will need to monitor Anna closely for signs of infection, which poses risks to both of you." The other option—nonintervention—would mean letting nature take its course.

When the doctors left the room, Anna and David were alone, engulfed in silence. Tears streamed down Anna's face as she clung to David. "How are we supposed to make this decision?" she asked, her voice trembling. "How can we choose what's right?"

David felt the weight of her words pressing down on him. Every fiber of his being wanted to protect both of them, but the path ahead was shrouded in uncertainty. "I don't know," he whispered. "But if there's a chance… we have to try."

Hours later, they informed the doctors of their decision: they would pursue an active approach. The team sprang into action. Anna received corticosteroid injections, and labor-slowing medications were administered. Every hour brought new checks—temperature readings, blood tests, monitoring for the faintest sign of infection.

Over the next three days, Anna and David lived on the precipice of hope and fear. Contractions came and went, sometimes subsiding, sometimes gaining strength. The medical team moved with precision, balancing intervention with vigilance. On the third day, labor could no longer be delayed. Anna's contractions intensified, her body preparing for what lay ahead. David never left her side, gripping her hand as each wave of pain washed over her.

Finally, their baby was born—tiny, fragile, and fighting to breathe. The room erupted in controlled urgency as the neonatal intensive care unit (NICU) team moved swiftly to stabilize the newborn. The baby was immediately intubated and connected to a mechanical ventilator to support breathing, as the underdeveloped lungs struggled to function on their own. The initial assessment yielded an Apgar score of 3 at 1 min. With rapid intervention, including ventilation and intensive monitoring, the score improved to 5 at 5 min, a small but hopeful sign of stabilization.

In the NICU, every breath remained a battle. The baby lay in an incubator, surrounded by tubes and monitors that tracked every heartbeat, oxygen level, and vital function. Anna and David visited as often as they were allowed, whispering words of love through the small openings in the incubator. They marveled at the tiny fingers that wrapped around theirs with surprising strength, cherishing each precious moment in the face of overwhelming uncertainty. The days blurred together, a mix of cautious optimism and ever-present fear.

On the seventh day, the nightmare returned. The baby developed necrotizing enterocolitis (NEC), a severe condition affecting the intestines of preterm infants. The medical team worked tirelessly, but the infection spread rapidly.

The doctors' voices were calm yet resolute. "We've done everything we can," they said gently. "Now it's time to prepare."

Anna and David held their baby close, a fragile life they had hoped to nurture and watch grow. As they cradled their child, they felt every faint heartbeat and treasured the quiet moments of connection. There were no grand gestures or words—only a deep, quiet presence. They whispered their love, a love that would remain etched in their hearts forever. When the room finally fell silent, they stayed close, taking comfort in the knowledge that they had given their child every possible moment of care and connection.

In the days that followed, their home felt both achingly quiet and overwhelmingly full of reminders of their loss. Anna and David found themselves navigating a future that looked so different from the one they had imagined. Yet, even amid their grief, they held onto the solace that their baby had known care, warmth, and love. Slowly, they began to find strength in the small acts of remembrance and the enduring impact of their child's brief but meaningful presence in their lives.

1.2 Introduction

The birth of a child is a moment of joy and wonder for most families, yet for those whose babies are born extremely prematurely, it becomes a race against time. Infants born before 28 weeks of gestation, classified as extremely low gestational age newborns (ELGANs), face an uphill battle for survival. Their organs are critically underdeveloped, and even with modern medical care, their chances of thriving without severe complications remain low.

Despite decades of advancements in neonatal care, extreme prematurity continues to carry high rates of mortality and long-term disability. This reality underscores the urgent need for transformative innovations that go beyond incremental improvements in existing technologies.

1.3 The Challenges of Extreme Prematurity

Each year, about 15 million babies are born prematurely worldwide. Among them, nearly one million will not survive. For those who do, the journey often comes with significant health challenges, including chronic diseases, neurodevelopmental impairments, and respiratory complications. The burden of prematurity is not only emotional but also economic. Estimated global costs associated with preterm births likely exceed $100 billion annually, encompassing direct medical expenses, long-term care, and broader societal impacts.

1.4 Respiratory Challenges

One of the most immediate dangers facing extremely preterm infants is respiratory distress syndrome (RDS). This condition arises because their lungs lack surfactant, a critical substance that prevents the collapse of alveoli during breathing. However, the issue goes deeper than surfactant deficiency. In infants born before 24–26 weeks, the lungs have not yet entered the saccular stage of development, where alveoli—the tiny air sacs responsible for gas exchange—begin to form. Instead, their lungs are in the canalicular stage, characterized by primitive airways and a lack of functional alveoli. This fundamental immaturity makes effective gas exchange nearly impossible, even with the best medical interventions.

Mechanical ventilation, a lifesaving necessity for these infants, often causes additional damage to their fragile lungs. High-pressure oxygen delivery can lead to bronchopulmonary dysplasia (BPD), a chronic lung condition that affects about 50% of ELGANs requiring prolonged ventilation. BPD not only prolongs oxygen dependency but also increases the risk of long-term respiratory complications and hospitalizations.

1.5   Neurological Vulnerabilities

The immature brain of a preterm infant is particularly vulnerable to injury. Intraventricular hemorrhage (IVH), or bleeding within the brain's ventricular system, occurs in about 25% of ELGANs. This condition often originates in the germinal matrix, a fragile area of the brain involved in neurodevelopment. Severe cases of IVH can result in permanent cognitive and motor impairments, including cerebral palsy.

Another common complication is white matter injury, which damages the brain's communication pathways. This condition affects 10–20% of ELGANs and can lead to significant developmental delays, including difficulties with coordination, learning, and sensory processing.

1.6   Cardiovascular and Gastrointestinal Risks

The cardiovascular system of extremely preterm infants is not fully prepared to support life outside the womb. Patent ductus arteriosus (PDA), a condition in which a fetal blood vessel fails to close after birth, affects about 50% of ELGANs and can cause heart failure and pulmonary overcirculation. Hypotension (low blood pressure), another common issue, can lead to inadequate perfusion of vital organs, further increasing the risk of damage.

The gastrointestinal system is also highly immature, making ELGANs susceptible to necrotizing enterocolitis (NEC), a life-threatening intestinal disease affecting about 7–10% of preterm infants. Survivors of NEC often face long-term complications, including bowel dysfunction and poor growth.

1.7   Infections and Immune Deficiency

The underdeveloped immune systems of ELGANs leave them highly susceptible to sepsis, a life-threatening systemic infection that affects nearly 20% of these infants. Infections not only increase the risk of mortality but also prolong hospital stays and complicate recovery.

1.8   The Limits of Current Interventions

While modern neonatal care has saved countless lives, it has reached a plateau in its ability to significantly improve outcomes for ELGANs. Over the past decade, survival rates for extremely preterm infants have increased modestly, yet the rate of survival without severe disabilities has remained largely unchanged.

Even with advancements like antenatal corticosteroids, exogenous surfactant therapy, improved ventilation strategies, and specialized NICU protocols, many infants still face lifelong complications. This stagnation highlights the inherent limitations of current technologies, which address symptoms rather than the root causes of prematurity-related complications.

For instance, while surfactant therapy has dramatically reduced the mortality associated with RDS, it cannot compensate for the lack of alveoli in infants born during the canalicular stage. Similarly, while mechanical ventilation keeps infants alive, it often exacerbates the very conditions it seeks to treat, such as BPD and IVH.

1.9   The Economic and Emotional Costs

The economic burden of prematurity is staggering. In the United States alone, annual costs are estimated at $26 billion, encompassing NICU care, surgeries, medications, and long-term therapies. For families, the financial strain is compounded by the emotional toll of caring for a child with complex medical needs. Parents of ELGANs often experience heightened levels of stress, anxiety, and depression, particularly as they navigate the uncertainty of their child's prognosis.

1.10   A Call for Revolutionary Solutions

Given the immense challenges faced by ELGANs and their families, it is clear that traditional approaches to neonatal care are insufficient. Incremental improvements in existing technologies are unlikely to yield significant gains. Instead, a paradigm shift is needed—one that reimagines how we care for extremely preterm infants.

The development of revolutionary technologies, such as the artificial placenta and artificial womb, represents a promising avenue for research and innovation. By mimicking the natural environment of the womb, these systems could provide the necessary conditions for continued growth and organ development, allowing preterm infants to bypass many of the complications associated with their early birth.

While these solutions are still in the experimental stage, they offer hope for a future where extreme prematurity no longer carries such devastating consequences. As research progresses, the potential to transform neonatal care and improve outcomes for the world's most vulnerable patients becomes increasingly tangible.

1.11 Conclusion

Extreme prematurity remains a formidable challenge in neonatal care, with high rates of mortality and long-term disability. Despite the strides made in recent decades, the current state of neonatal technology has reached its limits in addressing the root causes of complications. The urgency for innovation has never been greater. By pursuing revolutionary solutions that go beyond existing paradigms, we can aspire to a future where survival is not merely possible but accompanied by the promise of a healthy, thriving life.

2

Beyond the Boundaries: The Drive to Develop Babies Outside the Female Body

2.1 From Fear to Hope: Anna and David's Extraordinary Path to Parenthood

Ten years had passed since Anna and David first faced the challenges of extreme prematurity. The memories of that tumultuous time—neonatal intensive care unit (NICU) alarms, invasive interventions, and the ache of uncertainty—remained vivid, etched into their minds. Yet life had moved forward. Their child's short but meaningful life had left them changed, and they carried those experiences with them as they navigated the years ahead.

When Anna discovered she was pregnant again, the news evoked both joy and anxiety. The excitement of a new beginning was tempered by the shadow of their past experience. They not only knew the risks and possibilities, but they also knew how far technology had come. Advances in artificial womb technology and perinatal care offered hope that had once seemed unimaginable.

At their first consultation, the obstetrician addressed their concerns with empathy and optimism. "The technology today is very different from what you experienced ten years ago," she explained. "If complications arise, we have solutions that didn't exist then. Let's focus on supporting this pregnancy every step of the way."

But at 24 weeks, Anna's water broke unexpectedly, and once again, their world was turned upside down. This time, however, the options were different. The hospital staff acted swiftly and calmly, explaining the possibilities with a clarity that gave Anna and David a sense of control.

© The Author(s), under exclusive license to Springer Nature Switzerland AG 2025
G. Oei, *The Artificial Womb*, Copernicus Books,
https://doi.org/10.1007/978-3-031-85905-2_2

"The artificial womb technology has advanced significantly," the obstetrician said. "We've had remarkable success with it, and it's no longer limited to hospitals. If your baby is born prematurely, we can set up the system in your home, allowing you to experience the pregnancy in a familiar and peaceful environment."

The prospect was surreal but comforting. They agreed to proceed, knowing it offered their baby the best chance. When labor began, the process felt surreal. The delivery room was filled with focused activity as their tiny baby was delivered and carefully transferred into a specialized transferbag, maintaining the warmth and amniotic-like environment. The transition from Anna's womb to the artificial system was seamless, ensuring the baby remained undisturbed by the change.

Soon, the artificial womb—a transparent biobag filled with synthetic amniotic fluid—was set up in the corner of Anna and David's living room. Compact, self-sustaining, and equipped with advanced correctional systems, it maintained the perfect environment for their baby's growth. A technical physician at the hospital remotely monitored the setup, ensuring every detail—from oxygenation to nutrient delivery—remained precisely calibrated.

For Anna and David, the experience was transformative. The hum of the artificial womb became a comforting presence, a reminder of the life it nurtured. They could watch their baby's movements on a connected monitor and feel the tiny kicks and rolls through a haptic-feedback artificial abdomen that transmitted their baby's activity to Anna's belly.

"It's incredible," Anna whispered one evening, her hand resting on the dome of the artificial womb. "To feel the baby moving, to know everything is safe—it's more than I ever dared to hope for." David, seated beside her, added softly, "It feels like we're part of this journey in a way we weren't before."

The artificial womb offered more than a physical space; it brought peace. Unlike the chaotic intensity of a traditional neonatal intensive care unit (NICU), their home became a haven. The baby was free from invasive tubes, mechanical ventilation, and the stress of harsh lights and sounds. Instead, the artificial womb provided a fluid environment that supported lung development and minimized the risks of infection and organ damage.

As weeks turned into months, Anna and David grew closer to their baby. They read stories aloud, played music, and marveled at ultrasound images of tiny fingers curling and eyelids fluttering. The medical team, freed from constant crisis management, devoted their time to guiding Anna and David through every milestone with patience and care.

At the end of three months, their baby reached a pivotal moment—the transition to life outside the artificial womb. The doctors carefully orchestrated the transfer, ensuring the baby emerged fully developed and strong enough to breathe *independently. The anticipation was overwhelming, and when Anna finally cradled her child in her arms, tears streamed down her face.*

"You're here," she whispered, her voice unsteady. "You're really here." David leaned in, his hand resting gently on their baby's back. "We've waited so long for this moment," he said softly. "And it's perfect."

As they settled into life as a family, Anna and David reflected on the incredible journey they had taken. The artificial womb had not only nurtured their baby but had given them the chance to experience pregnancy in a way that felt natural and connected, despite the technology's complexity.

Yet, they were also acutely aware of the broader implications of the technology. "It's amazing what's possible now," Anna said one evening. "But it makes you think about what this means for the future—for other families, for society."

David nodded. "This technology makes you rethink so much about pregnancy and parenthood. It's not just about science—it's about how we approach life and what matters most."

For Anna and David, their journey was one of hope and determination. It showed how innovation, combined with compassion, could open new possibilities for families like theirs. But it also highlighted the ethical questions that come with such advancements—questions society will need to address as these technologies continue to evolve.

2.2 Introduction

The field of obstetric care faces one of its most pressing challenges with extreme prematurity. Babies born so early that their organs are underdeveloped confront a precarious start to life, highlighting the urgent need for innovative solutions.

2.3 The Artificial Womb

A groundbreaking innovation that holds promise is the artificial uterus. This technological marvel could transform neonatal care by offering a lifeline to those born too early. The artificial womb replicates the nurturing environment of a natural womb, providing a haven for continued growth and development outside the mother's body.

Picture a state-of-the-art, transparent chamber, where a fetus is cradled in a fluid-filled environment, simulating the amniotic sac (Fig. 2.1). In this controlled space, conditions are meticulously tailored to mimic those of a natural

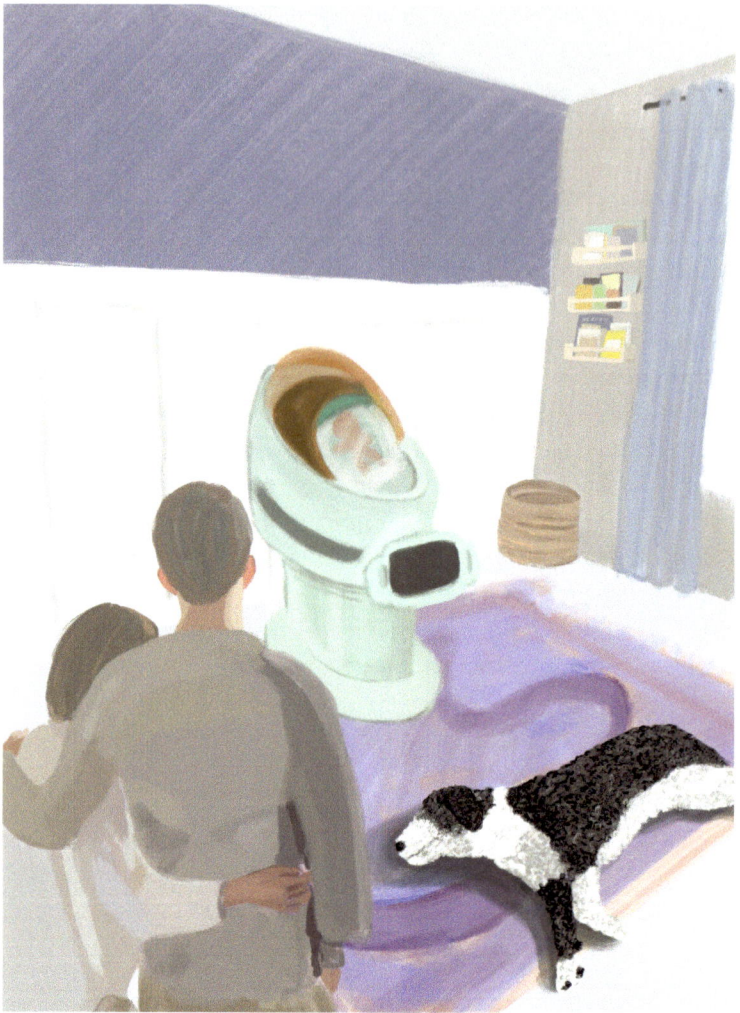

Fig. 2.1 A glimpse of tomorrow: A couple watches over their prematurely born baby in an artificial womb, illustrating the potential future of neonatal care. Their dog sleeps peacefully nearby, grounding this extraordinary moment in the comforts of everyday life

womb, providing warmth, nutrition, and respiratory support essential for premature babies. The implications of this technology are profound, offering hope for infants with underdeveloped lungs, hearts, and brains who currently face high risks of death or lifelong disabilities. An artificial uterus can provide a safe, stable environment for these infants to continue their development until they are strong enough to survive in the outside world.

The benefits of artificial uteruses extend beyond immediate medical advantages. They have the potential to reduce health risks and complications associated with traditional pregnancies, particularly those leading to premature births. By offering a controlled environment, these devices can improve outcomes for both mothers and babies, reducing the incidence of long-term health issues. Moreover, the artificial uterus could represent a significant advancement for individuals and couples facing fertility issues, offering a new path to parenthood by bypassing certain biological limitations and providing a controlled environment for successful gestation.

2.4   Ethical Implications

However, the ethical implications of this technology cannot be overlooked. It raises profound questions about the nature of birth, the definition of motherhood, and the ethical considerations of creating life outside the human body. These are questions that require careful, thoughtful consideration by the scientific community, ethicists, and society. Approaching this innovation with a sense of responsibility and ethical awareness is crucial. This technology is still in its early stages, and while its potential is immense, rigorous testing, ethical debate, and collaborative research are essential. Co-creation with patients is pivotal in developing cutting-edge healthcare technologies, ensuring that innovations are patient-centric, ethically sound, and practically viable.

The growing interest in developing babies outside the female body reflects a complex interplay of medical, social, and technological advancements. Medically, the development of artificial uteruses offers a potential solution for those who cannot conceive naturally or carry a pregnancy to term. Traditional neonatal care methods often reach their limits with extremely preterm births due to the underdevelopment of vital organs. For instance, a child born before the third trimester typically has underdeveloped lungs, and introducing air under pressure into these immature alveoli poses significant risks. Similarly, the immature gastrointestinal system of a preterm infant can lead to complications like necrotizing enterocolitis, which can be fatal. The artificial womb aims to create conditions that mimic the natural uterine environment, allowing the preterm infant to continue developing as if it remained in the mother's womb.

Maternal health is another critical factor. Complications such as preeclampsia, gestational diabetes, or the dangers associated with premature births pose significant health risks to both mother and child. For instance, women who have experienced hypertension during pregnancy are at increased risk for both coronary artery disease and atrial fibrillation later in life. An external gestational environment could potentially mitigate these risks, ensuring the health and safety of both.

2.5   Societal Perspective

From a societal perspective, the development of babies outside the female body addresses issues of gender equality and personal choice. It allows individuals and couples, regardless of gender or sexual orientation, to experience parenthood. This technology can democratize reproductive rights, offering an equitable choice for all who wish to become parents.

However, this journey is not without its ethical complexities. The concept of ectogenesis challenges traditional views on pregnancy, motherhood, and the sanctity of life. It brings to the fore questions about the bond between mother and child, the societal roles of women, and the very nature of human reproduction. As this new era unfolds, it is imperative to balance the potential of this technology with thoughtful consideration of its ethical and societal implications. The role of the medical community extends beyond the boundaries of practice into the realms of moral responsibility and social advocacy.

2.6   Ectogenesis

Ectogenesis has been a topic of both scientific inquiry and speculative fiction for decades. One of the earliest and most influential literary explorations of this concept can be found in Aldous Huxley's dystopian novel *Brave New World*, published in 1932. In this futuristic society, traditional reproduction is replaced by the artificial breeding and conditioning of humans in "hatcheries and conditioning centers." Huxley's portrayal of ectogenesis reflects deep societal and ethical concerns that resonate even today as biotechnology advances.

In 1958, a significant development occurred when researchers successfully grew a mouse embryo outside the womb for the first time, marking a milestone in reproductive biology. This breakthrough fueled apprehensions similar to those depicted in Huxley's work. The possibility of ectogenesis raises questions about the ethical, social, and psychological impacts of separating human reproduction from the human body. This debate reflects our ongoing struggle to balance the potential benefits of such technologies with their profound moral and societal implications.

The birth of the first "test-tube baby," Louise Brown, in 1978 was a pivotal moment in reproductive medicine. This achievement was the result of the pioneering work by Robert Edwards and Patrick Steptoe, driven by the desire to help couples struggling with infertility. Edwards' contributions to this field were recognized with the Nobel Prize in Physiology or Medicine in 2010, underscoring the profound impact of in vitro fertilization (IVF) on reproductive medicine. This innovation not only opened new possibilities for treating infertility but also raised important ethical and societal questions about assisted reproductive technologies. As with the development of IVF, the advancement of artificial uteruses will likely follow a similar pattern, where technological progress precedes ethical and regulatory frameworks.

In vitro fertilization (IVF) represented a groundbreaking moment in reproductive medicine. However, the medical achievement was immediately accompanied by intense ethical debate, with questions and concerns raised about the moral implications of creating human life outside the body. The introduction of IVF marked a significant shift in how society understood conception, parenthood, and the role of medical technology in these intimate areas of human life.

2.7 Ethical Debate on IVF

At the heart of the ethical controversy surrounding IVF was the issue of the human embryo. For the first time, embryos could be created, manipulated, and even frozen outside the human body. This sparked fierce opposition from religious and ethical groups, particularly those who believed that life begins at conception. They argued that if an embryo was a form of human life, then the process of creating "extra" embryos—some of which would inevitably be destroyed—was morally unacceptable. This led to heated discussions about whether embryos should be granted legal and moral status as persons and how they should be treated within the scientific process.

Many critics, particularly from religious organizations such as the Catholic Church, argued that IVF was a form of "playing God," intervening in the natural process of conception. They feared that if science could manipulate reproduction in this way, it would pave the way for further, more troubling forms of genetic manipulation. The idea of human life being engineered or created outside the natural order seemed to cross a dangerous line, raising concerns about where such scientific advancements might lead. Would IVF be the first step toward genetic engineering or selecting certain traits in future children, or perhaps even to the creation of "designer babies"?

Beyond the moral and philosophical questions, IVF also raised concerns about its impact on society. In many traditional views of family, the biological connection between parents and children played a key role in identity and inheritance. IVF, by enabling conception outside of sexual reproduction, disrupted these longstanding norms. Some questioned how children born through IVF might be treated or perceived in society. Would they be seen as "less natural" or even stigmatized? Although these fears largely proved unfounded, they were prevalent during the early years of IVF's introduction.

There was also concern about the social inequities that IVF could create. As the procedure was initially expensive and available only to a select few, many feared that access to this revolutionary technology would be restricted to wealthy families, exacerbating social inequality. For many, the prospect of a technology that could help overcome infertility was bittersweet—promising for those who could afford it, yet frustrating for those who could not.

Despite these concerns, the success of IVF gradually shifted public perception. Overtime, as more babies were born through IVF and grew into healthy children, the initial fear and suspicion began to subside. Studies have shown that children conceived through IVF are generally as healthy as those conceived naturally, with only a slight increase in the risk of certain conditions, often related to prematurity or multiple births due to the transfer of multiple embryos.

Today, over ten million babies have been born through IVF, and the technology has become a mainstream option for couples struggling with infertility. While the early ethical debates highlighted valid concerns, society has largely embraced IVF as a positive development, offering hope to millions of families worldwide.

2.8   Ethical Debate on ICSI

In the 1990s, a new advancement in reproductive technology emerged—intracytoplasmic sperm injection (ICSI). This technique allowed for the injection of a single sperm directly into an egg, offering hope to men with very low sperm counts or poor sperm motility, who otherwise might not have been able to father a child. ICSI rapidly became a successful method for treating male infertility, but like IVF, it raised its own ethical questions.

While ICSI was seen as an extension of IVF, the ethical concerns surrounding it were distinct in certain ways. One of the major issues with ICSI was the more direct manipulation of the reproductive process. Critics argued that by bypassing natural selection at the level of sperm fertilizing the egg, ICSI might allow genetic defects or fertility problems to be passed on to future generations. This raised concerns about the long-term consequences for children conceived through this method, though overtime, most studies have found that ICSI children have similar health outcomes to those conceived through traditional IVF or natural conception.

Despite these fears, ICSI was celebrated for providing a solution to male infertility, which had been a major hurdle in reproductive medicine. In many cases, men who would never have been able to father a child were now given that opportunity. This shift in the possibilities of reproduction was monumental, but again, it raised concerns about how far technology should go in overcoming natural reproductive barriers. Would this lead to even more invasive forms of intervention in human reproduction?

Much like IVF, ICSI also led to discussions about how such technologies might affect societal notions of parenthood and biological legacy. For example, if a man with genetic infertility was able to father a child through ICSI, would his child inherit the same infertility? Some ethicists questioned whether it was responsible to bypass natural selection to this extent, potentially propagating genetic issues that would otherwise have been filtered out. However, for many, the ability to create families where it was previously impossible outweighed these concerns.

As with IVF, the fears surrounding ICSI have diminished overtime as the technique has become more widespread. Studies on the health of children born through ICSI have largely been reassuring, with no significant long-term health problems directly associated with the procedure. Today, it is estimated that over six million babies have been born through ICSI, and the technique is now a common part of fertility treatment, particularly for couples where male infertility is a factor.

2.9   Health Outcomes of IVF and ICSI Children

The long-term health of children born through IVF and ICSI has been a topic of intense research over the years. Initially, there were concerns that these children might face higher risks of birth defects or other health problems due to the artificial nature of the conception process. However, most studies have shown that children born through IVF and ICSI are generally as healthy as those conceived naturally. Some slight increases in risks have been noted, particularly in cases where multiple embryos are transferred, leading to higher rates of prematurity and low birth weight. These factors, however, are more related to the circumstances of multiple births rather than the technologies themselves.

In the case of ICSI, concerns about passing on genetic causes of male infertility remain, but they have not materialized into widespread issues. While there may be some increased risk of genetic infertility in male offspring, this has not been a significant factor in most cases. Overall, both IVF and ICSI have been deemed safe, with millions of healthy babies born worldwide, thanks to these technologies.

The introduction of IVF and ICSI fundamentally changed the landscape of reproductive medicine, offering hope to millions of couples who previously had little chance of conceiving. While these technologies were initially met with ethical debates over the manipulation of life and the potential long-term consequences, they have since become accepted and widely used methods for overcoming infertility. As science continues to advance, it is likely that new technologies will emerge, each bringing its own set of ethical considerations. However, the lessons learned from the introduction of IVF and ICSI have paved the way for a more informed and thoughtful approach to balancing the promises of medical technology with the moral questions they raise.

In conclusion, developing a physiological alternative to the incubator through the artificial uterus is a promising frontier in neonatal care. It offers hope for premature infants and addresses significant medical, ethical, and societal challenges. As this technology advances, it is essential to approach it with a balanced perspective, ensuring that it is developed responsibly and ethically.

3

Ethical Considerations on Ectogenesis

3.1 The Two Paths of Ectogenesis: A Story of Promise and Complexity

Emma and Daniel had spent years trying to conceive. Their journey had taken them through every fertility treatment imaginable, each one ending in heartbreak. Finally, when they were about to give up, they heard about a revolutionary new option—ectogenesis, the growth of an embryo entirely or partially outside the womb. It offered a solution not just to their infertility, but to the heartbreak of premature birth, a reality that had touched their extended family. The technology not only held promise, but it also came with uncertainties and ethical considerations they needed to confront.

Sitting across from their fertility specialist, Emma and Daniel listened intently. "There are two paths to consider," the doctor explained. "Partial ectogenesis focuses on premature infants, supporting them in an artificial womb after a natural pregnancy reaches a critical, but still precarious, stage. This can dramatically improve survival rates and reduce complications. Complete ectogenesis, on the other hand, involves creating and nurturing life entirely outside the womb, from conception to birth."

Emma glanced at Daniel before speaking. "Can you tell us more about the partial approach?" she asked, her tone thoughtful. The doctor acknowledged her question with a slight smile and began outlining the transformative impact partial ectogenesis was having on neonatal care. In cases of extreme prematurity, traditional neonatal intensive care units (NICUs) often faced insurmountable challenges. Babies born too soon struggled with underdeveloped organs, high risks of

© The Author(s), under exclusive license to Springer Nature Switzerland AG 2025
G. Oei, *The Artificial Womb*, Copernicus Books,
https://doi.org/10.1007/978-3-031-85905-2_3

infection, and a harsh world of invasive tubes and mechanical ventilation. "In contrast," the doctor continued, "an artificial womb provides warmth, nutrition, and a stable, regulated environment for the baby's continued development. It mimics the natural uterus, allowing for growth without the physical trauma and stress of traditional care."

Emma imagined what it would be like to see her baby growing safely in an environment that replicated the womb. There would be no invasive attachments, no relentless alarms, and less anxiety over breathing difficulties. It was a hopeful vision. "This could give babies like my sister's preemie a chance," Daniel whispered, thinking of the nephew who had not survived.

But there was another side to ectogenesis, one that went deeper than the promise of better outcomes for preterm infants. "Complete ectogenesis is where things become more complex," the doctor said gently. "Creating a life entirely outside the human body challenges everything we know about pregnancy, birth, and parenthood. It raises questions about when life begins, how we define personhood, and what rights someone gestated this way would have. The technology has the potential to help people like you, but society is still grappling with what it all means."

Emma and Daniel left the clinic deep in thought. In the weeks that followed, they explored every aspect of ectogenesis. They spoke with parents who had used partial ectogenesis for their preterm infants, who described the joy and relief of watching their babies grow and thrive without the constant fear of NICU complications. They learned that many of these children had fewer long-term health issues, thanks to the controlled, nurturing environment that supported their development during the most critical weeks.

But they also delved into the ethical debates surrounding complete ectogenesis. What would it mean for a child to be born without a mother's touch, without the experience of being carried in the womb? Would society view these children differently? Would they have the same rights and protections? Discussions with ethicists and legal experts revealed the moral and legal gray areas that remained unresolved. What defined "viability" when life could be sustained from the earliest stages outside the womb? And how should they refer to an individual who had never been "born" in the traditional sense?

Emma and Daniel found themselves at the crossroads of promise and uncertainty. Partial ectogenesis offered clear medical benefits and a more straightforward path, but the potential of complete ectogenesis was harder to navigate. It had the power to change society's approach to reproduction, fertility treatments, and even what it meant to be a family. Yet, it also posed questions that went beyond the scientific and medical questions about identity, connection, and ethics.

In the end, Emma and Daniel decided to pursue partial ectogenesis if needed. They would continue to try for a natural pregnancy, but the knowledge that this technology was available, ready to offer a lifeline if their baby came too soon, brought them a sense of peace. As they moved forward, they recognized that their story was just one of many. The development of ectogenesis had the potential to transform lives, but it also demanded careful thought and responsible stewardship. As Emma said to Daniel one evening, "It's not just about us. It's about what this means for everyone—today and in the future."

Across society, the journey toward understanding and integrating ectogenesis would require open dialogue, co-creation of policies, and thoughtful reflection. The technology's potential was immense, but it could not be embraced blindly. Balancing medical benefits with societal values, and respecting the complexities of human experience, would be key to ensuring that ectogenesis truly served humanity in the way it was meant to.

3.2   Introduction

Ectogenesis, whether partial or complete, marks a significant advancement in addressing major medical challenges like infertility and premature birth. Partial ectogenesis, which focuses on supporting prematurely born infants, and complete ectogenesis, the development of an embryo entirely outside the body from conception to birth, offer different possibilities for medical intervention. However, they also raise complex ethical, legal, and social questions that must be addressed before they can be widely implemented (Fig. 3.1).

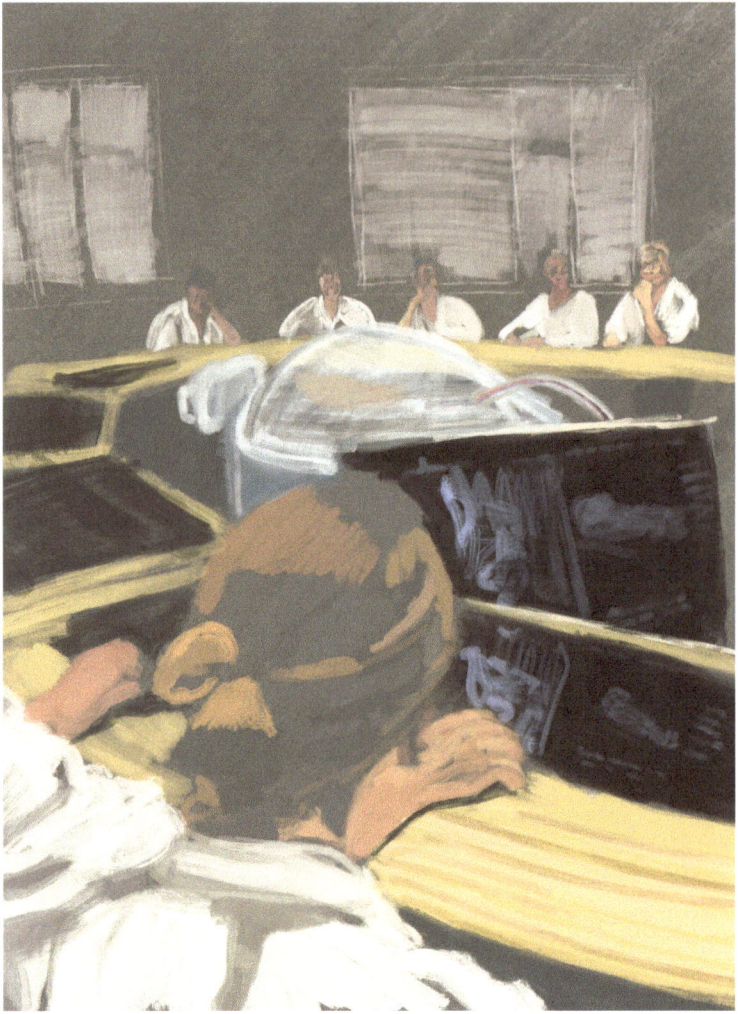

Fig. 3.1 Deliberating the future: navigating the moral landscape of ectogenesis

3.3   Partial Ectogenesis

Partial ectogenesis offers groundbreaking potential for improving the survival and development of preterm infants. By mimicking the natural environment of the womb more closely than current incubators, partial ectogenesis could reduce the risks of long-term health complications commonly associated with premature births, such as respiratory problems, cerebral palsy, and cognitive delays. This technology could allow extremely premature babies to grow in an environment that more closely replicates the natural conditions of gestation, giving them a better chance at healthy development. Premature birth remains a significant global health challenge, with millions of infants born prematurely each year, many of whom face lifelong complications or mortality. Partial ectogenesis holds great promise in addressing this widespread issue by creating safer and more regulated conditions for the maturation of these vulnerable infants.

3.4   Complete Ectogenesis

On the other hand, complete ectogenesis—gestation entirely outside the body—presents a more speculative future. It could provide an alternative pathway to parenthood for individuals who cannot carry a pregnancy to term due to medical conditions, the absence of a uterus, or other health risks. While the technological advancements in this area are notable, complete ectogenesis has a much narrower medical application compared to partial ectogenesis, which addresses a more pressing and widespread medical need. Complete ectogenesis also raises more profound ethical questions about the nature of pregnancy, childbirth, and the bond between mother and child. If gestation occurs entirely outside the human body, it challenges traditional concepts of pregnancy and parenthood, prompting concerns about the commodification of childbirth and the reduction of pregnancy to a mechanical process.

3.5   Ethical Concerns

Ethical concerns surrounding both partial and complete ectogenesis are not only focused on the potential medical benefits but also on the broader societal implications. For partial ectogenesis, the question revolves around how far medical intervention should go in sustaining life outside the womb. Should we embrace technologies that extend the boundaries of neonatal care, or should we accept certain natural limits? For complete ectogenesis, the debate becomes even more complex, as it fundamentally challenges the biological and emotional connections traditionally associated with pregnancy and birth. Ethicists like Joanna Verweij, Elselijn Kingma, Chloe Romanis, and Nick Colgrove have all contributed to this discussion, raising essential questions about the moral, legal, and societal implications of these technologies.

Verweij and colleagues have outlined a comprehensive framework for the ethical development and introduction of artificial womb technologies. Their approach emphasizes the importance of public discussion, ensuring that the language used to describe these technologies is accessible and understandable to everyone. This transparency is essential for gaining public acceptance and ensuring that these technologies are introduced in ways that align with societal values. Verweij also stresses the importance of designing technologies with ethical considerations in mind from the outset, ensuring that they reflect the values of the communities they are intended to serve. Additionally, she emphasizes that research involving these technologies must be conducted with the highest ethical standards, with informed consent and a thorough understanding of the potential risks and benefits by all participants.

Philosophers and bioethicists like Kingma have explored the potential redefinition of pregnancy that might arise from the advent of artificial wombs. Kingma's work highlights how ectogenesis could transform our understanding of gestation, shifting it from a biological process tied to the mother's body to something that could be externalized and managed by technology. This shift raises questions about parental rights and responsibilities, particularly in cases where pregnancy might be outsourced to an artificial womb. Romanis has contributed to this discussion by introducing the term "gestateling," a unique entity created by ex utero gestation, which she argues is neither a fetus nor a newborn. This new category challenges our existing legal and ethical frameworks, as it represents an entirely new stage of human development.

Colgrove has critiqued Romanis's position, arguing that gestatelings should be treated the same as newborns, regardless of their developmental environment. He asserts that the differences between a gestateling and a newborn are not significant enough to warrant different legal or moral status. This debate touches on fundamental questions about personhood and when human life should be granted full moral consideration. Romanis counters by emphasizing that gestatelings are distinct entities, having not undergone the traditional process of birth, and therefore, their moral status may differ from that of a newborn.

These debates are not merely theoretical, they have practical implications for how we define birth and personhood in the context of ectogenesis. Traditionally, birth has been understood as the moment when a baby transitions from the womb to independent life, typically marked by the initiation of breathing. However, a gestateling does not undergo the same biological processes as a newborn, raising questions about whether it should be considered "born" at all. Romanis argues that gestatelings, especially those who have developed through partial ectogenesis, should still be considered "unborn" because they have not completed the full biological process of birth. Colgrove, on the other hand, believes that if a gestateling can survive independently outside an artificial womb, it should be granted the same status as any newborn.

One of the most critical questions in this debate is how to define the moment of birth for children who have spent part or all of their gestational period in an artificial womb. In partial ectogenesis, the transition from the artificial womb to independent life aligns more closely with traditional definitions of birth, as the fetus has already spent time developing in the natural womb. However, in complete ectogenesis, where the entire gestation occurs outside the body, the moment of birth becomes less clear. Is it when the child exits the artificial womb, or when it begins to function independently?

Legal systems will need to adapt to these new realities. Currently, many legal definitions of birth are tied to the physical separation of the baby from the mother's body and the initiation of independent breathing. These criteria may not apply in cases of ectogenesis, particularly complete ectogenesis, where the child may never have been connected to a mother's body in the traditional sense. Lawmakers and ethicists must work together to develop new definitions that account for these technological advances while protecting the rights and dignity of the child.

3.6   Terminology

One of the other challenges in discussing ectogenesis is the terminology we use to describe the entities involved. Romanis's term "gestateling" has sparked debate over whether we need a new word to describe a fetus developing in an artificial womb. Other proposed terms include "fetonate," a blend of fetus and neonate, and "perinate," which refers to the perinatal period surrounding birth. However, the most logical and descriptive term might simply be "fetus in an artificial womb." This terminology is clear and easily understood, directly linking the developmental stage of the entity (fetus) with its unique environment (artificial womb). It avoids the confusion that new terms like "gestateling" might introduce, while still acknowledging the distinct nature of ectogenetic development.

This clarity in terminology is essential as we navigate the ethical and legal questions surrounding ectogenesis. By using precise and descriptive language, we can ensure that discussions about ectogenesis remain accessible to the public and avoid unnecessary confusion. The term "fetus in an artificial womb" allows us to communicate effectively about this new form of development while respecting the established stages of human gestation.

In conclusion, ectogenesis, whether partial or complete, holds significant potential for addressing infertility and premature birth, but it also raises complex ethical, legal, and societal challenges. Partial ectogenesis offers a promising solution for premature infants, potentially improving their survival rates and long-term health outcomes. Complete ectogenesis, while still speculative, could provide an alternative path to parenthood for those unable to carry a pregnancy. However, the introduction of these technologies requires careful consideration of their broader implications. Legal definitions of birth, parental rights, and the moral status of fetuses in artificial wombs will all need to be reexamined. The most logical and clear terminology to describe these entities is "fetus in an artificial womb," as it directly communicates both the developmental stage and the unique environment involved. As we move forward, it is essential to engage in open, transparent discussions that involve all stakeholders—patients, medical professionals, ethicists, and the public—to ensure that ectogenesis is developed and implemented in a way that aligns with societal values and protects the dignity and rights of all individuals involved.

4

Historical Perspectives on the Beginning of Life in Art

4.1 The Secrets Within: The Birth of Horus

The desert air was dry and heavy as the excavation team descended into the tomb. Dust lingered in the flickering torchlight, and every cautious step stirred the sand that had lain undisturbed for centuries. The discovery of the Tomb of Ramses VI was an achievement already being whispered about in academic circles, but nothing could have prepared them for the secrets that lay within.

Bruno, a junior archaeologist on his first major expedition, held his breath as the heavy stone door to the burial chamber creaked open. For months, he had sifted through rubble, meticulously cataloging fragments of pottery and tools. But now, standing at the threshold of history, he felt the weight of the moment settle on his shoulders.

The torchlight spilled into the vast chamber, revealing walls alive with color and detail. Figures of gods and goddesses danced across the stone, their forms etched with care and reverence. Among the depictions of Isis, Nephtys, and Osiris, one central image caught his eye: a radiant scene of the birth of Horus, surrounded by celestial symbols and intricate hieroglyphs. Bruno stepped closer, his heart pounding as he raised his torch higher to illuminate the carvings.

There, in vivid detail, Isis cradled the unborn Horus within her womb, her hands encircling him protectively. The cosmic imagery surrounding her seemed to pulse with meaning. Bruno could almost hear the ancient whispers of the priests who had once guarded this sacred space. "It's like … they've captured the moment of creation itself," he murmured to his colleague, his words filled with wonder.

The hieroglyphs told a story of cosmic balance and renewal. The Egyptians believed that every birth mirrored the creation of the universe—a sacred act where

G. Oei, *The Artificial Womb*, Copernicus Books, https://doi.org/10.1007/978-3-031-85905-2_4

chaos was overcome, and order restored. In the carvings, the developing fetus was rendered with remarkable anatomical accuracy, and Isis's womb was surrounded by spiraling symbols that represented the cycles of life and death.

As Bruno moved further into the chamber, he paused, his gaze lingering on a carving of a crocodile standing behind a man. The details were vivid, yet the identity of the figure eluded him. He wondered aloud, "Could this represent Sobek, the god of the Nile? Or perhaps… Tawaret?" The latter thought made him smile. Tawaret, the hippopotamus goddess of childbirth, was rarely depicted in tombs like this, but her symbolic presence often transcended the physical. She embodied protection and the cycles of life, much like the broader themes of the tomb itself.

While Bruno found no clear depiction of Tawaret among the murals, her influence seemed to linger in the atmosphere of the chamber. "Even without her image here," he mused, "her essence feels present. This tomb is steeped in the same reverence for life and birth that she represents."

The days turned into weeks as Bruno and the team meticulously documented the murals. One image, in particular, captured his imagination—a depiction of the Earth as a floating island, encircled by primordial waters. The comparison to a fetus within the amniotic sac was unmistakable. The circular Achet, or horizon, represented both the boundaries of the known world and the protective enclosure of the womb.

Bruno lingered in the chamber long after his colleagues had left for the day. He sat with his notebook open, tracing connections between the scenes on the walls and the stories they told. The ancient Egyptians had viewed birth not just as a biological event but as a cosmic act, deeply connected to the cycles of creation and renewal. In his mind's eye, Tawaret stood quietly among the other deities, unseen yet ever present, a silent protector watching over the mysteries of life.

On the final day of their excavation, Bruno stood before the carvings one last time. The sun had begun to dip below the horizon, casting a golden glow into the chamber. "A guardian of beginnings," he murmured, feeling a deep respect for the ancient beliefs that had imbued these walls with such profound meaning. As he stepped back into the desert's fading light, he carried with him not just the artifacts and notes but a newfound reverence for the enduring mysteries of life and the timeless quest to understand them.

4.2   Introduction

The journey of art and science reminds us of the importance of thoughtful discourse in the face of rapid technological change. Throughout history, the depiction and understanding of pregnancy and the beginning of life have evolved significantly, reflecting the prevailing societal values, scientific knowledge, and ethical considerations of each era. From the earliest cave paintings that celebrated fertility and the mysteries of birth, to the intricate sculptures and religious iconography of ancient civilizations, art has always played a crucial role in how humanity perceives and reveres the origin of life. The Renaissance period, with its fusion of art and expanding scientific inquiry, marked a profound shift in our understanding of human anatomy and reproduction, setting the stage for more informed and nuanced discussions about pregnancy and the inception of life. As we moved into the modern era, advancements in medical science and technology, coupled with changing social norms, further transformed our views and practices surrounding childbirth and prenatal development. The depiction of pregnancy in contemporary art, influenced by feminist movements and bioethical debates, continues to challenge and expand our perceptions. This chapter takes you on a journey through these historical milestones, highlighting key moments and artistic expressions that have shaped our current understanding of pregnancy and the beginning of life. It explores how these developments have gradually led us to contemplate the concept of ectogenesis—the artificial womb and the possibility of gestating life outside the human body.

The future of ectogenesis, much like its artistic and scientific precursors, will be shaped not just by technological capability but by ethical considerations, societal values, and the ongoing dialogue between science and art. Art remains a vital companion to science, not only reflecting humanity's hopes and fears but also actively shaping the conversation about our future and the new frontiers of human reproduction. By examining the intersection of art, science, and societal values, we gain a deeper appreciation for the complexities and possibilities that lie ahead in the realm of human reproduction.

4.3   The Timeless Fascination with Birth

Since the dawn of time, the miracle of birth has captivated the human imagination, weaving a thread of awe and reverence through the fabric of our existence. This profound fascination transcends mere biological curiosity, touching the very core of what it means to create, to nurture, and to continue the cycle of life. It is a story as old as humanity itself, written in the heartbeats of countless generations and echoed in the diverse expressions of cultures across the globe. In the hushed whispers of ancient caves, our earliest ancestors left their marks—enigmatic figures and symbols etched into stone and painted on walls, celebrating the enigma of creation. These primal artworks, like the Venus figurines with their exaggerated forms, were not just representations of the physical act of birth but symbolized a deeper understanding of the role of fertility and maternity in the continuity of life. As we travel through history, we see a reverence for birth expressed in the myths and religions, in art and literature, and in the quiet expressions of sculpture and painting. Each era, each culture, each artist, and each storyteller bring a unique perspective to the narrative of birth, adding layers of meaning and interpretation that reflect the prevailing beliefs, knowledge, and sentiments of their times.

4.4   Prehistoric Beginnings: The Cradle of Artistic Expression

Our odyssey into the artistic representation of birth and fertility begins in the remote corridors of prehistory, where the nascent stirrings of human creativity first sought to capture the essence of life's genesis. In this era, unadorned by the written word, our ancestors communicated their awe and understanding of creation through the universal language of art. The Venus figurines, such as the famed Venus of Willendorf, stand as silent yet eloquent witnesses to this early reverence for fertility and maternity. Dating back to around 25,000–30,000 years ago, these figurines are found across parts of Europe, particularly in regions like modern-day Austria, France, Italy, Germany, and Eastern Europe, each one a small, tactile sculpture carved from stone, bone, or ivory. Their exaggerated forms—ample breasts, rounded bellies, and full hips—are not mere artistic whimsy but deliberate emphasis on the aspects of the female form associated with childbirth and fertility. They symbolize, perhaps, the prehistoric understanding of the woman's role as a bearer of life, a tangible connection to the mysterious and powerful forces of nature that governed existence.

Equally compelling are the prehistoric cave paintings, such as those in Lascaux, France, and Altamira, Spain. While not explicitly focused on maternity or childbirth, these paintings often include symbols and figures that suggest a reverence for the cycle of life. Animals in various stages of growth, scenes that hint at the rhythms of nature, and the occasional depiction of human figures amid these natural tableaus speak of a deep-seated recognition of the interconnectedness of all life forms. In these earliest artworks, we see the foundational threads of humanity's enduring fascination with birth. These creations were more than mere depictions; they were an integral part of the ritual and spiritual fabric of prehistoric societies. They represent humanity's first attempts to grapple with the profound mysteries of where we come from and how life perpetuates itself—questions that continue to intrigue and inspire us to this day. As we trace this artistic journey through the ages, these prehistoric beginnings remind us that the wonder of pregnancy and the miracle of birth have always been central to the human experience. They laid the groundwork for the countless artistic explorations to come, each adding depth and perspective to our understanding of one of life's most enigmatic processes.

4.5 Ancient Civilizations: Mythology and Maternity

As we journey from the primordial art of prehistory into the realms of ancient civilizations, we encounter a rich tapestry of mythology and iconography centered around childbirth and fertility. These themes, deeply ingrained in the cultural fabric, found expression in the art of ancient Egyptian, Greek, and Roman societies.

4.6 Egyptian Civilization: The Divine Feminine

In ancient Egypt, the goddess Isis epitomized the ideals of motherhood and fertility. She was often depicted in art and sculpture as a nurturing mother, symbolizing both literal and metaphorical rebirth. The myth of Isis resurrecting her husband Osiris and subsequently conceiving their son, Horus, positions her as a figure of fertility and regeneration. The depictions of Isis with Horus on her lap, found in numerous temple reliefs and sculptures, resonate with the theme of protective and nurturing motherhood. In ancient Egyptian mythology, Horus was often invoked for protection and as a guardian, which by extension includes safeguarding the health of mothers and their newborn children. Horus's birth story is significant in Egyptian mythology. He was born posthumously after his father, Osiris, was murdered and dismembered by Seth, and his mother, Isis, reassembled Osiris's body and conceived Horus. Isis then had to hide Horus in the marshes to protect him from Seth until he was old enough to claim his throne. This story underscores themes of miraculous birth, survival, and the triumph of good over evil, which could be symbolically significant in the context of birth.

4.7 The Birth of Horus

Dr. B.H. Stricker (1910–2005) was a Dutch Egyptologist and historian of the religions of Antiquity. He was not only an expert in the Egyptian language, but he had also delved into Hebrew, Sanskrit, Old Persian, Arabic, and Berber, with the purpose of filling the gaps in the cultural history of Egypt by studying contiguous areas and contemporary cultures.

In his seminal work, the birth of Horus, he demonstrates that the "Embryologic Treatise" found in the burial chamber of Ramses VI, through its cosmological imagery of world creation, reveals the ancient Egyptians' attempts to understand the development and evolution of a human baby from conception to birth (Fig. 4.1).

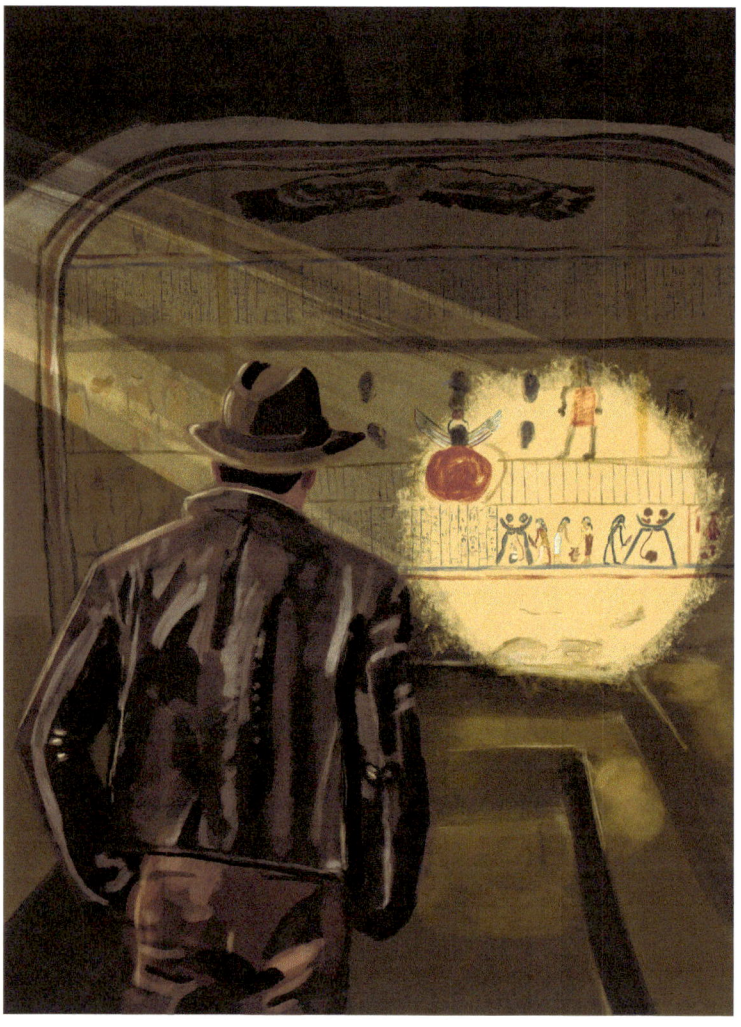

Fig. 4.1 Unveiling the past: exploring the depiction of life in the Tomb of Ramses VI

All ancient civilizations deeply explored the origins of the world, focusing on cosmology—the study of the universe's structure and history—and embryology—the study of an embryo's development. This fascination with origins formed the bedrock of their original philosophical concepts, centered around ideas of divine existence. Each entity was viewed as the result of a process, an evolution, mirroring the embryonic development of a human in the womb. This concept led ancient people to draw parallels between cosmology and embryology, perceiving the macrocosm of the universe and the microcosm of human development as reflections of each other. Thus, individual ontogeny, the development of an organism, was seen as a recapitulation of cosmic creation.

This belief also influenced cultural metaphors, linking cosmic events to human experiences. For example, the relationship between heaven and the Earth was likened to that of man and woman, with the fertilizing rain promoting growth as a woman's labor produces a child, mirroring the soil's fertility. Similarly, the annual flooding of the Nile, vital for fertilizing Egypt's lands, was compared to the act of fertilization itself, positioning the entire region of Egypt metaphorically as a uterus. Such metaphors extended to deities like Osiris and Isis, who were likened to a bull and a cow, representing the fertility and life-giving forces of nature.

Before the discovery that the Earth was spherical, the ancient Egyptians conceptualized the world as a flat disc encircled by an ocean, much like a vast river. Surrounding this body of water was a circular mountain range, which they referred to as Achet—literally translating to "the horizon" in hieroglyphics. Above this cosmic circle-shaped mountain, the sky was imagined as a lid sealing the world. Beyond this boundary lay only the abyss and chaos, rendering the entire world akin to a cavernous entity (Fig. 4.2).

Therefore, the world itself is akin to a macrocosmic womb. Within this conception, the cosmic circle-shaped mountain, Achet, is symbolized or personified by the goddesses Isis and Nephtys. Horus, the son of Isis, represents all that the Earth produces and sustains: the people, animals, and vegetation. In later interpretations, the Earth is depicted as a floating island within this cosmic cave, supported by a series of columns (Fig. 4.3).

In this view, the Earth is likened to a baby, reminiscent of Horus in the womb of his mother, as depicted through hieroglyphs. Macrocosmically, it represents the primal sea—the primeval waters encircling the Earth like a river, analogous to the amniotic fluid surrounding the unborn in a mother's womb. Just as a baby first sees the light of the world at birth, originally Horus was brought forth by Isis and Osiris. Similarly, each day, the sun emerges from the vulva of Nut, the Goddess of Heaven, ascending from the horizon like a bird—Horus emerging from the uterus like a falcon.

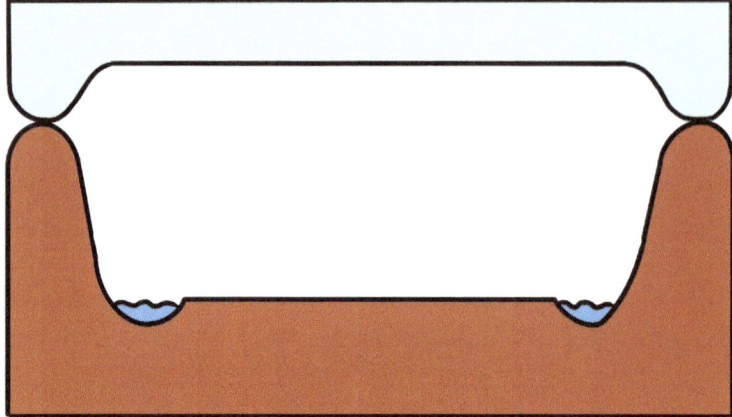

Fig. 4.2 The world cavity resembling an empty womb

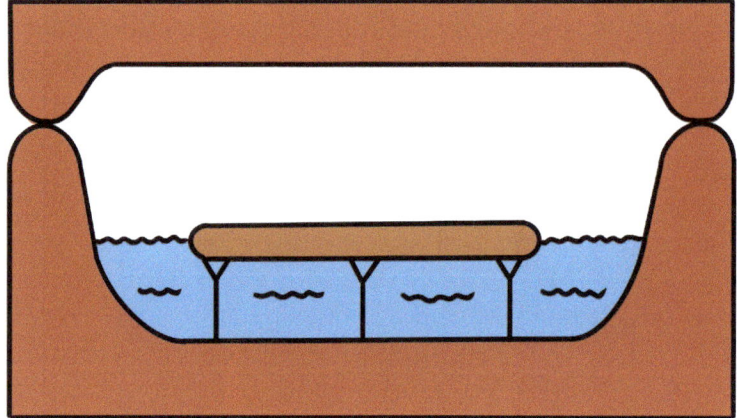

Fig. 4.3 The world cavity as a pregnant womb

The symbol of this daily rebirth is the lotus, a type of water lily that rises from the depths of the primal sea, its stem representing the umbilical cord, unfolding its petals at the surface to bloom. At the dawn of creation, the Sun God Ra spontaneously arose from these primeval waters, seated atop the primeval lotus like a newborn baby.

Stricker's most significant work involves his analysis of the Egyptian "Book of the Earth," or "Book of Aker," found in the burial chamber of Ramses VI, from the twentieth Dynasty around the twelfth century BCE. Stricker interprets this text as "The Embryological Treatise," culminating in the birth of a baby (Fig. 4.4).

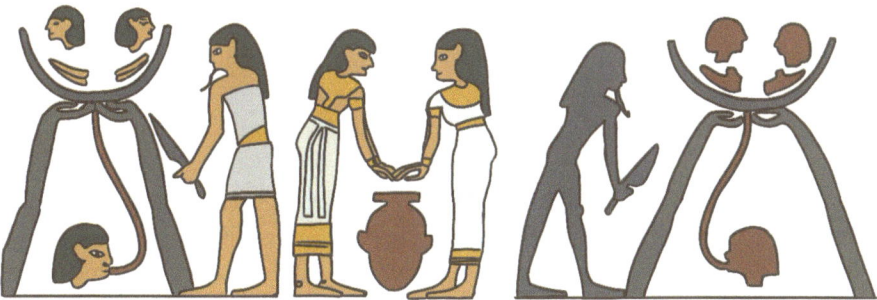

Fig. 4.4 Womb with fetus connected to placenta. Tomb of Ramses VI twelfth century before Christ

The pairs of arms on the left and right side of the picture represent the uterus. The ribbons with heads beneath them symbolize the umbilical cord and its attachment, the placenta. Above, on the left and right, are bowls containing two human heads—one pair facing each other, the other turned away—and two symbols that, according to the text, represent body parts. The moment of birth is depicted, as the arms, by their posture, suggest pushing away rather than receiving. The newborn is contained within both bowls. The two heads in the bowl are the child itself and the placenta, connected and facing each other on the right, and turning away and separating on the left. The separation of the two, as well as the general separation of the fetus and uterus, is presumably accomplished by the figures with knives. The entire scene is arranged in the form of the hieroglyph for Akhet, which represents the birth of the sun from the horizon (Figs. 4.1 and 4.2). This implies that the groups on the left and right, the pairs of arms, symbolize the mother, and the central group represents the embryo. This central group is depicted as a vessel in the shape of a heart sheltered by the two goddesses Isis and Nephtys, the two mothers. This heart vessel should, therefore, be considered as the fetus. The embryo is united with and nourished by the mother as long as the umbilical cord is intact. Macrocosmically, this representation indicates the birth of the sun god from the primordial waters. In Greek, the placenta is called "deuteron," meaning "second," which also refers to the moon in relation to the sun. In this interpretation, the two heads in the bowl symbolize the sun and moon, born apart at the zenith of the sky. The embryo, which was only potentially an individual in the mother's body and lived there like a fish in water, becomes actual through birth. In the ancient world, this is expressed using the symbol of the lotus. This plant grows in the water of the pond, representing the primordial waters and potential matter. Once matured, it emerges to the surface, blooms, and symbolizes both essence and act. There is a fundamental distinction between act and potential. Birth fundamentally occurs through opposition: what was closed opens; what was open closes. The umbilical cord, which nourished the child in the womb, would kill it outside if not cut. The amniotic fluid, which was life-giving for the embryo, would cause the child to suffocate. In Egyptian symbolism, the umbilical cord was regarded as a snake. Just as the snake was born from the Earth, so the umbilical cord is from the mother. The embryo kills the umbilical cord by piercing the membranes with its head, which belong to the snake's body. By its birth, the child overcomes inherent evil. Macrocosmically, this victory is akin to the daily rise of the sun. The boundary between potential and act lies between the elements of water and air. Actualization occurs at the moment when the embryonic state gives way to breathing. This Egyptian approach to the moment of ensoulment was also held by the Chaldeans, inhabitants of classical Mesopotamia, the Greek philosopher Plato, and the Roman-Phoenician philosopher Porphyrius. It is, therefore, the air alone that actualizes and imparts the soul.

Tawaret, the hippopotamus-shaped goddess, held a prominent role in ancient Egyptian belief as the protector of mothers and children. Her image, often depicted as a composite of a pregnant hippopotamus, a crocodile's tail, and a lion's limbs, symbolized strength, fertility, and protection. She was particularly revered as a guardian deity during pregnancy and childbirth, a time fraught with peril in the ancient world.

Tawaret's importance lay in her ability to ward off evil spirits and ensure the safe delivery of children. She was often portrayed holding the sa symbol, signifying protection, and standing by magical wands or amulets used in birthing rituals. As a household deity, her likeness appeared on everyday objects such as pottery and beds, signifying her constant vigil over domestic life. Beyond her protective nature, Tawaret was linked to the concept of rebirth and regeneration, her association with the Nile's fertile waters paralleling the life-giving amniotic fluid of the womb.

4.8   Greek Civilization: Deities of Birth

In ancient Greece, childbirth and fertility were under the patronage of specific deities, each representing different aspects of pregnancy and birth. Artemis, often portrayed as the goddess of childbirth and virginity, was invoked by Greek women for a safe delivery. The duality of her being a virgin and yet a protector of childbirth reflects the complex Greek views on femininity and maternity.

Hippocrates, often referred to as the "Father of Medicine," did not explicitly define the exact moment when life begins in the way contemporary debates might frame the issue such as the moment of conception, birth, or the first breath. However, his works and the Hippocratic Corpus—a collection of texts attributed to him and his followers—offer insights into how life and the process of birth were understood in ancient Greece.

4.9 Key Points from Hippocratic Views

1. *Embryological development*: The Hippocratic texts describe the development of the fetus in the womb, noting stages of growth and development. These writings suggest an understanding that the fetus grows and develops progressively, indicating an ongoing process of "becoming" rather than a single moment marking the start of life.
2. *Birth process*: In Hippocratic writings, the process of birth is considered to be the culmination of pregnancy, involving the fetus emerging from the womb. This process is crucial and is treated with various medical interventions to aid the health of the mother and the child.
3. *First breath*: While the Hippocratic texts focus extensively on the physical and medical aspects of childbirth, including the cutting of the umbilical cord and the care immediately following birth, they do not explicitly pinpoint the definitive moment life begins. However, the act of breathing is certainly recognized as critical for the survival of the newborn, marking its functional independence from the mother.

4.10 Cultural and Philosophical Context

In broader Greek thought, including philosophical and mythological traditions, the first breath often held significant symbolic weight, associated with the soul entering the body and the beginning of independent life.

Throughout the millennia, humanity has been deeply captivated by the mysteries of birth and the continuation of life, a fascination that has consistently found expression in art. The journey begins in ancient civilizations, where fertility and childbirth were regarded not merely as biological processes but as divine gifts, intricately tied to the cosmos and the gods. The Romans, inheriting much from their Greek predecessors, held these themes at the center of their cultural and religious life. Fertility deities, like Venus, became symbols of both love and the endless cycle of life. Roman society viewed birth and motherhood not only through a personal lens but also as vital to the very fabric of their civilization. The legacy of family, lineage, and the transfer of power was often celebrated in Roman art, with themes of maternity and fertility serving as a bridge between the mortal world and the divine. Birth was both a personal triumph and a communal event, anchoring the present to both the past and the future.

Moving through the epochs, we see how the portrayal of birth in art evolved in tandem with the values and priorities of the time. The Middle Ages brought a shift in focus toward the spiritual significance of maternity, particularly through the figure of the Virgin Mary. No longer was the mystery of birth viewed primarily through a biological or even cultural lens, but as a sacred event orchestrated by divine will. Mary's depiction in the Nativity scenes of medieval art was not just a representation of motherhood but a powerful symbol of purity, faith, and the miracle of life itself. She became a vessel for hope, with the birth of Christ symbolizing salvation for all humankind. These portrayals emphasized the theological importance of birth, grounding maternity in a larger narrative of spiritual redemption.

As the Renaissance swept across Europe, a profound transformation occurred in the way artists engaged with the human body, and by extension, with the concept of birth. This era, with its revival of classical ideals and new-found enthusiasm for scientific inquiry, marked a pivotal shift from the symbolic to the empirical. Figures like Leonardo da Vinci became obsessed with uncovering the hidden mechanics of the human form. His anatomical studies, particularly his famous sketches of fetuses in utero, revealed an unprecedented understanding of the body's inner workings (Chap. 6, Fig. 6.1). These drawings were not only groundbreaking for their scientific accuracy but also for the way they bridged the gap between art and science. In this fusion of disciplines, da Vinci and his contemporaries challenged long-held perceptions of birth as a purely mystical event, presenting it instead as a marvel of human biology that could be observed, studied, and understood. The Renaissance was a period of immense intellectual curiosity, where artists began to depict pregnancy and birth with a newfound realism. Gone were the abstract or strictly symbolic portrayals; in their place were images grounded in the real, physical experiences of human life. This change not only reflected advancements in scientific knowledge but also mirrored a broader cultural shift. The Renaissance view of the human body, pregnancy, and birth was a celebration of humanity itself—a recognition that these experiences, though deeply personal, were also universal. This shift laid the groundwork for later explorations of birth in art, which would continue to evolve as society's understanding of the human body expanded.

As the Renaissance gave way to the Baroque period, the portrayal of maternity took on a more dramatic and emotional tone. Baroque artists were masters of using light, shadow, and texture to evoke deep emotions, and this is evident in the subtle ways they suggested pregnancy and birth. While many Baroque works did not explicitly depict pregnancy, artists used other elements—gestures, poses, and settings—to convey the emotional weight of motherhood. The body language of women in these artworks often suggested fertility or maternity, whether through the positioning of their hands or the way their clothing subtly emphasized the curves of a pregnant belly. The emphasis was not so much on the physical act of childbirth but on the emotional and psychological depth that surrounded it. In many ways, this period marked a shift from the intellectual to the emotional, reflecting the changing nature of society's relationship with birth and family.

As time passed, artists continued to evolve their exploration of motherhood, reflecting broader cultural and philosophical changes. The Rococo period, with its light, playful style, often depicted intimate domestic scenes where maternity was hinted at through subtle details—a cradle in the background or a woman gently resting her hand on her stomach. The emotional depth of earlier periods gave way to a more romanticized, almost idyllic portrayal of life, where the emphasis was on the beauty and serenity of home and family life. Yet even in this more delicate, carefree period, the presence of pregnancy, though understated, remained a vital undercurrent, highlighting its timeless importance to human existence.

With the advent of the nineteenth century and the rise of Romanticism, the depiction of pregnancy and childbirth in art took on new meaning. The Romantic movement, with its emphasis on emotion, individuality, and the sublime, provided artists with a fresh lens through which to explore maternity. Paintings from this era often depicted motherhood with a sense of grandeur and personal emotion, capturing not only the physical reality of pregnancy but also its psychological and spiritual weight. As we moved from Romanticism into Realism, however, a new kind of depiction emerged—one that was focused on the raw, unvarnished truth of everyday life. Realist artists like Gustave Courbet sought to portray motherhood not in idealized or abstract terms but in all its messy, complex reality. Courbet's works on maternity, while less focused on the overt display of pregnancy, often evoked the emotional and physical tolls of motherhood, offering a more grounded, truthful exploration of this fundamental human experience.

This increasing focus on the emotional and physical realities of motherhood paved the way for artists like Gustav Klimt, whose work in the early twentieth century redefined how pregnancy and fertility could be portrayed. Klimt's use of rich colors and intricate patterns brought a new level of symbolism to maternity, while his willingness to depict the female body in all its sensuality and power challenged societal norms. His work reflected a growing acknowledgment of the complexities of female sexuality and the central role of women in the creation of life. Following in Klimt's footsteps, artists like Egon Schiele and Frida Kahlo pushed the boundaries even further, using their own experiences of pregnancy and miscarriage to create raw, deeply personal depictions of the female body and fertility. By the mid-twentieth century, the conversation around motherhood had expanded beyond personal or symbolic experiences. Artists began to explore pregnancy and birth through the lens of technology and social change, culminating in today's artistic explorations of ectogenesis—the development of life outside the womb. As reproductive technologies continue to evolve, artists like Mark Kostabi offer a modern perspective on maternity, blending the biological and technological in ways that challenge traditional views of motherhood. In Kostabi's *Recent Memory* (front cover), the faceless mother cradling her child transcends individual identity, becoming a universal symbol of care, protection, and the enduring bond between parent and child. The anonymity of the figures evokes a timeless quality, hinting at a future where the biological roles of mother and child might be redefined by advancements in artificial womb technology. Yet, amid such transformations, the emotional connection remains central and unbreakable. Interestingly, this depiction of a nurturing figure without distinct human features invites comparison to Tawaret, the ancient Egyptian goddess of fertility and childbirth. Tawaret, portrayed as a hybrid of a hippopotamus, a crocodile, and a lion, symbolized the ultimate protector of pregnancy and childbirth, combining the strength, resilience, and nurturing power of these creatures. Tawaret's form was not purely human, emphasizing her role as a guardian of life rather than a biological mother. Could Kostabi's faceless mother, cradling her child in a world shaped by evolving reproductive technologies, subconsciously echo this ancient archetype? Just as Tawaret embodied the forces of nature safeguarding the unborn, Kostabi's painting may reflect a modern parallel—pointing to a future where the essence of protection and nurturing transcends biology, while the core mission remains unchanged: to ensure that the child, whether in a womb or an artificial equivalent, is shielded and nurtured in every way possible.

Thus, *Recent Memory* subtly calls to both past and future—a reminder of humanity's enduring commitment to safeguarding life, while contemplating new ways in which we might continue to do so in an ever-changing world.

This merging of art and technology reflects a broader societal shift. As science brings us closer to the possibility of gestating life outside the human body, art becomes a critical tool for exploring the emotional, ethical, and social implications of such advancements. Just as ancient civilizations used art to grapple with the mysteries of birth, modern artists use their work to engage with the profound questions raised by technologies like ectogenesis. How will these advancements change our understanding of family, gender roles, and the value of life? Art, as it has always done, invites us to explore these questions, offering a space for reflection and conversation. In this new era, the dialogue between art and science is more important than ever. As technology continues to push the boundaries of what is possible in reproduction, art provides a platform for society to engage with these changes on a deeper, more human level. Through the centuries, art has served as a mirror to our evolving understanding of birth and motherhood—capturing not only the biological realities of life but also the emotional, ethical, and philosophical complexities that come with it. Today, art remains a vital tool for exploring the future of birth and the meaning of motherhood in a rapidly changing world.

5

A Bioreactor for Early Embryo Development

5.1 The Frontier of Life: Balancing Science and Ethics in Embryonic Development

In a state-of-the-art laboratory nestled within the walls of a renowned scientific institute, a team of dedicated researchers worked diligently. Their focus was on understanding the earliest stages of human life. The lab hummed with quiet intensity as bioreactors gently rotated, housing synthetic embryo models (SEMs) suspended in a nutrient-rich solution. These models, derived from stem cells, offered an unprecedented view into the complex and often mysterious processes that take place just after an embryo implants in the womb.

The scientists knew that they were standing on the precipice of groundbreaking discoveries. By observing the differentiation of cells and the formation of vital structures like the embryonic disc and extraembryonic tissues, they hoped to unlock new possibilities in treating fertility issues, understanding pregnancy disorders, and addressing congenital conditions. Yet, despite the promise of their work, they remained acutely aware of its boundaries. The goal was not to create life from scratch but to study the delicate, formative stages of development—an endeavor that demanded both precision and humility.

Central to their research was a bioreactor designed to simulate the conditions of the womb. It kept the developing SEMs in constant, gentle motion, ensuring even exposure to nutrients and oxygen. The bioreactor's sensors monitored key parameters like temperature and pH, allowing for real-time adjustments that maintained a stable environment. As one researcher noted during a quiet moment of reflection,

"We're not creating life—we're observing it. We're trying to understand what happens when life begins to take shape."

The models had yielded significant insights, particularly in mouse studies where stem cells organized into structures that mimicked the development of embryos after implantation. These breakthroughs, however, also raised questions that extended far beyond the lab. As the team worked to create human SEMs capable of replicating key developmental stages, they were keenly aware of the ethical implications that loomed over their research.

In another wing of the institute, a separate team focused on a related but distinct challenge: the development of artificial womb technology to support premature infants. For babies born too early to survive on their own, this technology offered a lifeline—a controlled environment that mimicked the womb's protective embrace. By maintaining optimal conditions for lung, heart, and organ development, artificial wombs could bridge the gap between extreme prematurity and full-term birth.

Yet, even as the researchers celebrated these advances, they faced questions that cut to the heart of what it meant to nurture life. The idea of complete ectogenesis—gestating a fetus entirely outside the human body—was a very distant and speculative concept, but it captured public imagination and stirred ethical debates. The researchers found themselves caught between scientific ambition and societal concern. Would society accept a world where humans were gestated in labs? How would this reshape concepts of parenthood, reproductive rights, and the nature of human existence?

One researcher paused during a long day of experiments, reflecting on these dilemmas with a colleague. "We have to be careful," she said. "The line between supporting life and creating it outside the body is thin. If we cross it, we need to understand the implications."

The ethical considerations were profound. If an embryo were to be gestated entirely outside the body, at what point would it gain moral status? How would society define the rights of a fetus in such a situation? These were not questions that science alone could answer. They required input from ethicists, policymakers, and the public. And while the researchers focused on practical applications like supporting preterm infants, they recognized the importance of engaging in open dialogue about the potential uses and limits of their work.

The legal landscape added another layer of complexity. Restrictions on human embryo research varied widely across countries, reflecting deep-seated concerns about human dignity and the potential misuse of reproductive technologies. Navigating these laws was as challenging as the science itself. The researchers knew that even if technology advanced, legal and ethical frameworks would shape its application. Without careful consideration, the risks of misuse or unintended consequences loomed large.

One of the most pressing concerns was the potential societal impact of artificial wombs. For centuries, the biological bond between mother and child had defined human experience. Would gestation outside the body alter that bond? Could parents choose ectogenesis to avoid the physical challenges of pregnancy, and what rights and responsibilities would they have over a fetus in such a scenario? These questions, complex and deeply personal, demanded thoughtful reflection.

As they continued their work, the researchers remained committed to transparency and ethical responsibility. They knew that public engagement was essential. Social media, films, and open forums could help demystify the science, encouraging meaningful dialogue and ensuring that advancements aligned with societal values.

In the end, the journey toward understanding early human development and supporting vulnerable infants was as much about ethics as it was about science. The researchers pressed on, aware of the delicate balance they had to maintain. Every discovery brought hope—but also a responsibility to ensure that their work respected human dignity, ethical standards, and the complexities of life itself.

5.2   Introduction

Researchers at the Weizmann Institute of Science, under the direction of Professor Jacob Hanna, are exploring the frontier of embryonic development outside the human body, a field that captivates many with its potential to reshape reproductive science. However, it is crucial to emphasize that their research focuses on early embryo development, not on the complete gestation of a fetus outside the womb, known as ectogenesis. While advancements in this area may raise questions about the feasibility of complete ectogenesis, the leap from early embryonic research to full artificial gestation remains speculative and far from current scientific aims.

5.3   Bioreactor to Support Early Embryo Development

Hanna's work, along with that of other leading researchers, addresses a specific and challenging phase of development: the period after the embryo implants in the womb. This phase is notoriously difficult to study due to ethical restrictions and technical challenges, as it involves complex structures and processes like the formation of the embryonic disc, yolk sac, and layers of tissues that sustain the developing embryo. The focus of this research is on creating synthetic embryo models (SEMs), primarily from stem cells, which replicate these postimplantation stages in a lab setting.

One of the pivotal tools in this research is a bioreactor designed to support early embryo development (Fig. 5.1). This bioreactor, central to Hanna's experiments, creates an environment that mimics some of the physical conditions of the womb. At its core, the bioreactor is a rotating system that gently keeps the developing embryo in motion, allowing it to float in a nutrient-rich solution. This environment ensures that the embryo is evenly exposed to essential compounds like amino acids, vitamins, glucose, and dissolved

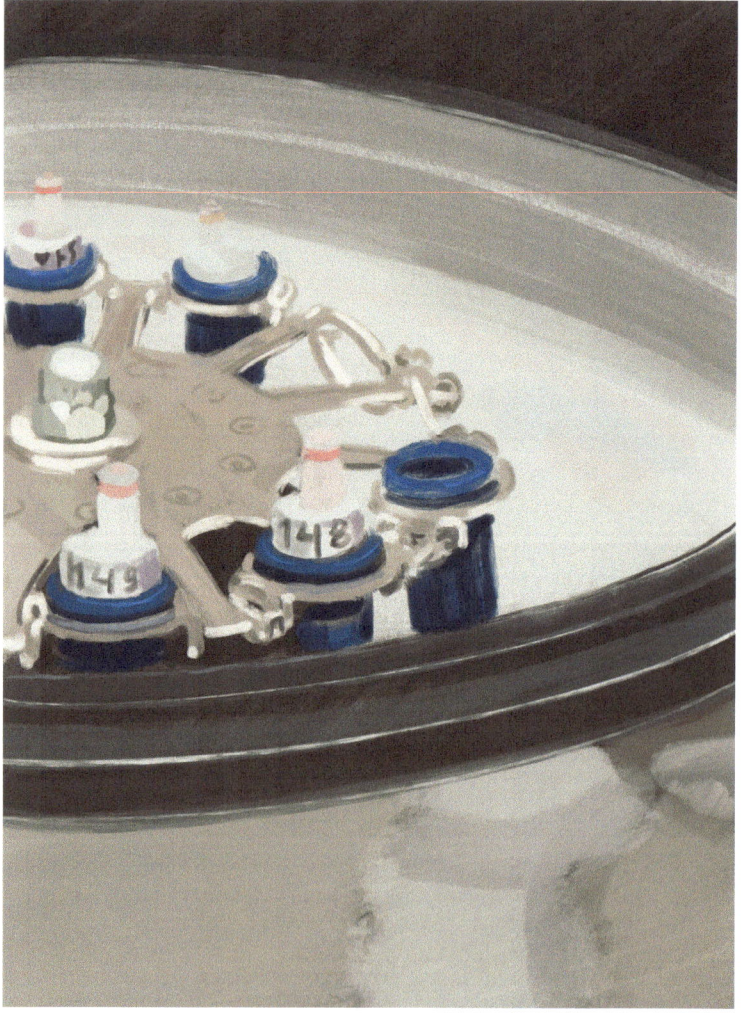

Fig. 5.1 Bioreactor for early embryo development

oxygen, which are critical for cellular respiration and energy production. The controlled fluid movement prevents the embryo from settling at the bottom or rising to the surface, ensuring uniform growth conditions.

The bioreactor is equipped with sensors and monitoring systems that track key parameters like temperature, pH, and oxygen levels in real time. These measurements allow for continuous adjustments to maintain a stable environment that mirrors the conditions of the natural womb. The goal of this bioreactor is not to replicate the entire pregnancy process but to study the very early stages of embryonic development. By observing how stem cells differentiate and organize into complex structures, researchers can gain unprecedented insights into the earliest phases of life.

Mouse models have been particularly promising, as mouse stem cells have successfully organized into structures that mimic the stages of development after implantation. These SEMs have allowed scientists to replicate early mouse embryo development up to mid-gestation, offering insights into this critical developmental period. Building on this success, Hanna's team has used human stem cells to create similar models. These human SEMs are made from unmodified naïve embryonic stem cells and replicate the key structures found in human embryos, such as the embryonic disc and extraembryonic tissues. The potential applications of this research are vast, including the possibility of better understanding and treating fertility issues, pregnancy disorders, and congenital abnormalities.

5.4   Gastrulation: A Cornerstone of Embryonic Development

Gastrulation is a critical phase in embryonic development, during which the three germ layers—ectoderm, mesoderm, and endoderm—are formed. These layers serve as the foundation for all organs and tissues in the body. This dynamic and highly coordinated process transforms the embryo from a simple blastula into a complex, multilayered structure. Despite its fundamental importance, studying gastrulation in humans has long been constrained by ethical considerations and the challenges of observing this process in vivo.

Professor Magdalena Zernicka-Goetz and her team at the University of Cambridge have pioneered research on gastrulation using synthetic embryo models (SEMs). These models mimic early embryonic stages, allowing researchers to observe gastrulation-like events in vitro. By demonstrating how stem cells can self-organize into structures resembling early embryos, Zernicka-Goetz's work provides unprecedented opportunities to study cell lineage specification, differentiation, and early organ formation in a controlled environment. These insights are invaluable for understanding normal development and the potential causes of congenital disorders or early pregnancy loss.

Zernicka-Goetz's research extends beyond gastrulation to include the study of postimplantation stages using advanced SEMs. These models replicate key developmental events, offering a valuable alternative to natural human embryos while avoiding ethical complexities. By integrating cutting-edge imaging technologies and gene-editing tools, research teams have been able to observe and manipulate specific developmental pathways in real time. This approach not only enhances our understanding of normal development but also opens new avenues for studying the origins of developmental abnormalities.

A central feature of gastrulation is the formation of the primitive streak, a structure that signals the beginning of germ layer differentiation. In natural embryos, epiblast cells migrate and differentiate into ectoderm, mesoderm, and endoderm. These layers later develop into the nervous system, muscles, bones, and internal organs. SEMs developed by Zernicka-Goetz's team replicate these critical early events, providing a platform for detailed observation and controlled experimentation. This work has deepened our understanding of how disruptions during gastrulation can lead to developmental defects.

Gastrulation can be likened to a sophisticated form of origami: just as a flat sheet of paper is folded and shaped into a complex three-dimensional figure, the initially simple structure of the embryo is transformed into a multilayered organism with distinct cell types and structures. This intricate process sets the stage for all subsequent development, solidifying gastrulation as a cornerstone event in embryogenesis.

5.5   Limitations and Challenges

Despite the impressive progress in SEM research, significant knowledge gaps remain. Our understanding of dynamic cell lineage specification, differentiation, fate patterning, and morphogenetic tissue organization during early postimplantation development is still incomplete. These processes are highly complex and require precise spatial and temporal coordination, making them difficult to replicate in vitro.

Moreover, while current SEMs can mimic certain structural and functional aspects of natural embryos, they lack the full biological context provided by maternal tissues during natural pregnancy. Critical interactions between the embryo and the maternal environment, such as nutrient exchange and hormonal signaling, are challenging to replicate in a laboratory setting. Addressing these limitations will require further technological advancements and inter-disciplinary collaboration.

5.6 Artificial Placenta Artificial Womb Technology

At the other end of the spectrum, artificial placenta artificial womb (APAW) technology is being developed for a different purpose. These APAW systems are designed to support extremely premature infants—those born too early to survive without significant medical intervention—by providing a controlled environment that mimics the conditions of the womb. This technology has the potential to revolutionize neonatal care, improving survival rates and long-term health outcomes for these vulnerable babies. Artificial wombs for premature infants, however, are fundamentally different from the idea of growing a fetus from conception to birth. They are designed to provide short-term support during a critical phase of development when the infant's lungs, heart, and other organs are not yet fully functional, bridging the gap between extreme prematurity and full-term birth.

5.7 Ethical and Societal Implications

The notion of complete ectogenesis also challenges long-held societal views on pregnancy and reproduction. For centuries, the biological bond between mother and child has been a defining aspect of human life. The development of artificial wombs raises fundamental questions about this connection, potentially transforming how we understand parenthood, reproductive rights, and the family unit. Could parents choose to gestate their child outside the womb to avoid the physical and medical challenges of pregnancy? What rights and responsibilities would parents have over a fetus gestating in an artificial womb? How would society regulate and monitor the use of such technologies? These are profound questions that extend beyond the realm of science and into the heart of societal values and norms.

Another concern is the potential for reproductive technologies, such as artificial wombs, to be used for purposes beyond their original intent. As with any new technology, there is a risk that ectogenesis could be used to pursue controversial goals, such as genetic modification or the creation of "designer babies." This raises additional ethical concerns about how far society is willing to go in altering the natural process of human reproduction.

Therefore, it is crucial that any future steps toward ectogenesis are preceded by an open and transparent public debate. This discussion must involve not only scientists and ethicists but also the broader public. Social media, films, and other forms of media can play an important role in fostering this debate, helping to demystify science and engage society in meaningful discussions about the future of reproductive technologies. By encouraging public participation, we can ensure that these advancements are developed and implemented in a way that aligns with societal values and ethical standards.

In conclusion, while the rapid progress in early embryo development and artificial womb technology is remarkable, the idea of complete ectogenesis remains speculative and distant. The focus of current research is on improving our understanding of early development and providing support for premature infants, not on creating a system that could entirely replace natural pregnancy. As these technologies continue to evolve, it is essential that we proceed with caution, ensuring that ethical, legal, and societal concerns are thoroughly addressed before taking any further steps. Co-creation of ethical frameworks with input from the public, medical professionals, and policymakers will be crucial in navigating the complex landscape of reproductive technologies. Only through transparent dialogue and careful consideration, can we ensure that these advancements align with our shared values and serve the best interests of society as a whole.

6

The Artificial Womb for Premature Infants: Protecting the Fetus from the Outside World

6.1 A New Hope: From News to Reality

Julia and Daniel had longed for a child for years, and after several failed attempts, their dream was finally coming true. Julia was now 21 weeks pregnant, but their excitement turned to fear when she unexpectedly went into early labor. Sitting anxiously in the waiting room after a rushed hospital visit, they clung to each other, trying to make sense of what might come next.

Later that evening, as they sat silently in front of the television, a news story caught their attention. The headline read: "Breakthrough in Artificial Womb Technology Keeps Preterm Lambs Alive for Weeks." The report showed footage of tiny lambs suspended in clear, fluid-filled sacs, thriving outside a natural womb. The anchor explained how this experimental technology could one day revolutionize care for extremely premature infants.

Daniel turned to Julia, a glimmer of hope in his eyes. "Do you think this could help us? Maybe it's closer than we think."

Julia hesitated, her mind racing. "It sounds incredible, but … would it really be ready in time for us?"

6.2 Seeking Answers

The next morning, they scheduled an appointment with Dr. Lewis, their obstetrician. They hoped she could provide clarity on what they had seen in the news.

© The Author(s), under exclusive license to Springer Nature Switzerland AG 2025
G. Oei, *The Artificial Womb*, Copernicus Books,
https://doi.org/10.1007/978-3-031-85905-2_6

"We saw a report about artificial wombs keeping preterm lambs alive for weeks," Daniel began, as they sat down in Dr. Lewis's office. "Is that something that could help us if things get worse?"

Dr. Lewis offered a kind but measured smile. "I understand why that news might give you hope, and it's true—there have been remarkable advancements in artificial womb technology. Researchers have managed to keep preterm animals alive for extended periods, and it has opened up exciting possibilities. But it's important to know that what you saw is still in the experimental stage. It will take years of rigorous testing before we can safely use such technology in human medicine."

Julia nodded slowly. "So, what does that mean for us now?"

"Right now," Dr. Lewis said gently, "our best approach is to try to delay labor for as long as possible and ensure you and the baby receive the best care. We'll monitor you closely, and if preterm birth becomes inevitable, we'll use current neonatal intensive care methods, which have come a long way in improving outcomes for premature infants."

6.3   Understanding the Science

As they left the appointment, Julia and Daniel felt a mix of emotions—relief that they were in good hands, but also a lingering curiosity about the technology they had learned about. That evening, Daniel decided to do more research. He learned that artificial wombs are designed to replicate the conditions of the uterus, providing a sterile, temperature-controlled environment filled with artificial amniotic fluid. Nutrients and oxygen are delivered through an umbilical interface, and the system aims to reduce the complications often seen with traditional neonatal care, such as lung damage from mechanical ventilation.

Julia joined him, reading over his shoulder. "It sounds amazing," she said. "But it also seems like there's still a lot they don't know."

Daniel agreed. "Yeah, there's talk about the challenges—things like preventing infections, making sure the baby's organs develop properly, and figuring out how to transition the baby out of the artificial womb safely."

6.4   A Long Road Ahead

The next few weeks were filled with uncertainty. Julia remained on bed rest, and each day without further complications felt like a small victory. Despite the challenges, they found comfort in knowing that science was moving forward, even if it was not fast enough to help them this time.

One evening, as they sat together, Julia said softly, "Even if it can't help us now, maybe someday it will help other families. Maybe our baby's struggle will be part of a bigger story."

Daniel squeezed her hand. "And who knows? Maybe someday soon, no one will have to go through what we're facing."

6.5   Hope Beyond Today

Julia and Daniel's story highlights the delicate balance between hope and reality that many families face when confronting extreme prematurity. The promise of artificial womb technology is profound, but it is tempered by the understanding that scientific breakthroughs take time—time measured in years of trials, setbacks, and progress.

Their experience reflects the broader challenge of involving patients in research. For many parents, the immediate goal is clear: to bring their child safely into the world. Yet others, like Julia and Daniel, see the value in contributing to a future where science may change the story for families yet to come.

Would parents like Julia and Daniel want to be involved in shaping such research? Likely, yes—but with the understanding that their primary concern remains the health of their child. Involving patients in the development of technologies like artificial wombs can provide invaluable insights. Their experiences can guide priorities, ensuring that future solutions not only improve medical outcomes but also address emotional and psychological needs.

6.6   Looking Ahead

Julia and Daniel may not have benefited directly from artificial womb technology, but they found solace in knowing that the future held promise. The story of artificial wombs is not just one of technical innovation—it is about a shared vision for a world where extreme prematurity no longer means life-threatening uncertainty. Through global collaboration, rigorous research, and perhaps even patient involvement, that vision may one day become reality.

In the meantime, families like Julia and Daniel remain at the heart of the journey, reminding us why innovation matters: to give every child the best possible start in life.

6.7   Introduction

Even with the significant advancements in neonatal care over the past decades, the mortality and morbidity rates of extremely premature infants remain alarmingly high. These newborns, defined as those born before 28 weeks of gestation, face severe challenges due to their underdeveloped organs. Conventional treatments, while lifesaving, often bring about their own set of complications. This has driven the need for innovative solutions like the artificial placenta and artificial womb technology (Fig. 6.1).

The concept of an artificial placenta and artificial womb was pioneered over 50 years ago with the goal of recreating the natural fetal environment to support the development of these fragile infants. The idea was to create a system that mimics the physiological functions of a real placenta and womb, providing a stable environment for normal organ development.

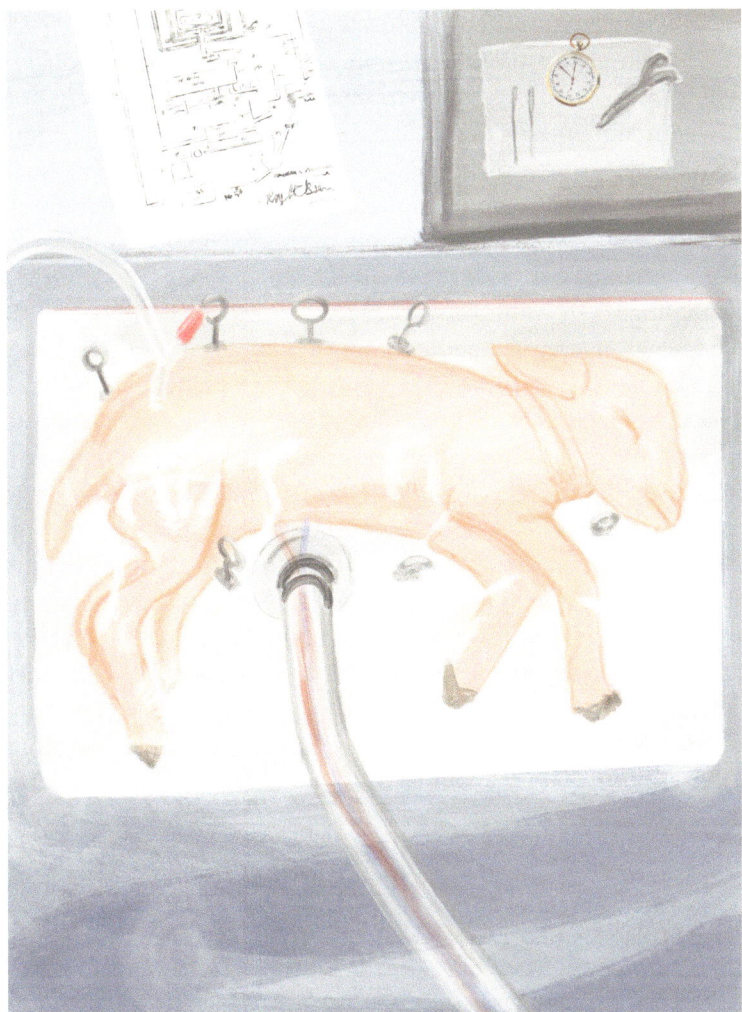

Fig. 6.1   The Biobag: A Pioneering Step in Perinatal Care

6.8   Japan's Advancements in Artificial Womb Technology

The real journey toward creating an artificial placenta and artificial womb began in Japan with Professor Yoshinori Kuwabara in the early 1990s. Kuwabara developed an "amniotic fluid bath" technique, immersing premature goat fetuses in a temperature-controlled, sterile fluid environment. This method closely mimicked the natural womb, providing a controlled setting for the fetuses to continue their development outside the mother's body. His innovative work demonstrated that it was possible to sustain fetal development for several weeks in an artificial environment, laying the foundational concepts that would inspire future advancements. Kuwabara's pioneering research showed that maintaining a womb-like environment could significantly impact the survival and growth of premature fetuses. His experiments opened the door to new possibilities in human neonatal care, suggesting that similar techniques could eventually be applied to support human preterm infants. Professor Kuwabara presented his work at the FIGO World Congress for Obstetricians and Gynecologists in Montreal in 1994 to an audience of 10,000 gynecologists. The reaction from the audience was one of admiration. If this could be applied to humans, it would mean a revolution for prematurely born children.

However, the road to success was fraught with significant challenges. One of the major problems encountered in Kuwabara's research was that the test animals frequently developed infections or suffered from brain hemorrhages. The root cause of these complications was twofold. First, the amniotic fluid could quickly become contaminated because the fetuses were housed in an open aquarium, exposing them to potential pathogens. Second, an external heart pump was used to circulate blood, necessitating the use of heparin to prevent clotting. Unfortunately, the fetuses were extremely sensitive to heparin, which often resulted in brain hemorrhages. These critical issues made it seem impossible to advance the technology further, causing the promising results of the early 1990s to be largely abandoned until new solutions could be found.

6.9 The Philadelphia Biobag: A Pioneering Step in Perinatal Care

The turning point came with Dr. Alan Flake and his team at the Children's Hospital of Philadelphia. Building on Kuwabara's foundational work, they developed the "biobag" system. This innovative artificial womb provided a sealed, sterile environment where extremely premature lambs, equivalent to 23-week-old human fetuses, could continue to develop in a manner similar to natural gestation. The biobag system addressed the two critical issues that plagued Kuwabara's experiments.

First, instead of an open aquarium, the biobag was a closed system that allowed the amniotic fluid to be continually refreshed, much like it is in a natural womb. This significantly reduced the risk of contamination and subsequent infections. Second, rather than using an external heart pump, the biobag system utilized the fetus's own heart to drive the extracorporeal circulation, known as the extracorporeal membrane oxygenation (ECMO). This approach required the development of an ECMO apparatus with a small blood volume and low resistance, as the fetal heart is very small and can easily become overloaded. By overcoming these two major hurdles, Flake's team did demonstrate that they were able to sustain fetal lambs from a developmental stage equivalent to 24 weeks in humans to 28 weeks for four weeks, suggesting that the biobag could support the growth and maturation of extremely premature human infants during this critical period.

Just three months after the Philadelphia group's publication, another team on the opposite side of the world presented similar findings. Dr. Haruo Usuda and Dr. Matthew Kemp, along with their colleagues at the Women and Infants Research Foundation and the University of Western Australia in Perth, published their research in the *American Journal of Obstetrics and Gynecology*. Their study focused on refining the ex vivo uterine environment therapy and testing its efficacy on preterm lambs.

6.10 The Perth Experiment

In Western Australia, a team of researchers embarked on an ambitious endeavor to refine artificial placenta technology, building upon earlier work done in other parts of the world. Their aim was to create a stable, long-term ex vivo environment for supporting extremely preterm fetuses. Recognizing the unique risks faced by preterm infants, such as infections and inflammation, the researchers focused on enhancing both the safety and physiological stability of their system.

Their approach shared several key elements with earlier systems, but it also featured crucial improvements. The artificial womb environment they developed was designed to maintain the fetus in a sterile, fluid-filled state, with synthetic amniotic fluid closely mimicking the conditions of the uterus. Special care was taken to ensure that blood flow through the umbilical vessels remained steady and that the risk of infection was minimized.

The results of their study were promising. Over the course of a week, the team successfully maintained seven out of eight preterm lambs in a stable condition. Key physiological parameters, including heart rate and blood pressure, remained within normal ranges, and there were no signs of infection or systemic inflammation. Postmortem analysis revealed that the lambs' growth and development were comparable to those of control animals kept in utero.

One of the most significant findings was related to lung development. Despite being supported entirely by extracorporeal oxygenation, the lambs exhibited normal lung growth. This outcome underscored the potential of the artificial placenta to support organ development without the complications typically associated with mechanical ventilation.

However, the study was not without its challenges. One lamb experienced complications due to a kink in the catheter, which temporarily interrupted blood flow and resulted in localized brain injury. This incident highlighted the need for further refinements in catheter design and positioning to prevent similar issues in future trials.

Overall, the Perth team's experiment represented a significant step forward in artificial placenta research. By demonstrating the feasibility of maintaining extremely preterm fetuses in a stable, growth-promoting environment for an extended period, they contributed valuable insights to the ongoing effort to translate this technology into clinical practice. Their findings offered hope that, with continued development, artificial placenta systems could one day improve outcomes for the most vulnerable preterm infants.

6.11 The Significance of Reproducibility

The nearly simultaneous and independently successful experiments conducted by these two groups were a pivotal moment for the field of neonatal care. The reproducibility of results by different teams in different parts of the world bolstered the credibility and promise of artificial womb technology. It demonstrated that this innovative approach could be reliably replicated, a critical step toward eventual clinical application in humans.

6.12 Looking Forward

These concurrent studies by Partridge, Flake, Usuda, and Kemp have paved the way for ongoing research and development in artificial womb technology. The collective findings underscore the potential to revolutionize care for extremely preterm infants, offering them a better chance at healthy development and reducing the long-term health complications associated with prematurity.

In Europe, researchers at the Eindhoven University of Technology have been making significant strides with their perinatal life support (PLS) system. The PLS system is an Artificial Womb and Artificial Placenta (APAW), filled with sensors and measuring instruments, based on digital twin methodology, providing decision support to the care team. Led by biomedical engineer Professor Frans van de Vosse, obstetrician Professor Guid Oei, and industrial designer Dr. Frank Delbressine, this interdisciplinary team is working to create a controlled, liquid-based environment that mimics intrauterine conditions for extremely premature infants.

What sets this group apart is their innovative use of a life-like simulation mannequin that closely resembles and reacts like a human fetus. To enhance the accuracy and responsiveness of the mannequin, they have integrated digital twin technology, creating a virtual model that mirrors the real-time physiological conditions of the fetus. This allows medical teams to practice complex procedures in a highly realistic environment, enabling better preparation for future clinical applications while eliminating the need for animal testing. The mannequin's realistic responses enable the team to anticipate and address potential challenges, ensuring that they are fully prepared for future human trials. By refining their techniques through this realistic simulation, they aim to deliver the safest and most effective care when transitioning to human experiments. The PLS system includes an artificial placenta that supplies oxygen and nutrients via the umbilical cord, advanced monitoring, and computational modeling to provide real-time clinical guidance. Their work represents a promising solution for bridging the gap between preterm birth and full-term development, combining expertise in cardiovascular biomechanics, industrial design, and perinatal care.

7

The Artificial Placenta: Feeding the Immature Infant

7.1 A Delicate Transition: The Promise and Challenge of the Artificial Placenta

The neonatal intensive care unit (NICU) hummed with the quiet efficiency of a world dedicated to saving lives. Lina sat by Noah's incubator, her hand resting on the plexiglass surface. Her baby, born at 26 weeks, lay surrounded by the tangle of tubes and wires that were keeping him alive. Each beep of the monitor felt like both a reassurance and a reminder of how fragile his life was.

Dr. Elena Moreau entered, clipboard in hand but her focus entirely on Lina. "We've been carefully monitoring Noah," she began, her tone calm and measured. "His oxygen levels are dropping, and his lungs aren't responding well to ventilation. We're reaching the limits of what conventional care can do."

Lina's throat tightened. She had hoped Noah's struggle would ease after the first 48 hours. "What does that mean?" she asked.

Dr. Moreau pulled up a chair. "There's a technology we can use—a kind of artificial placenta. It's not the same as an artificial womb; it doesn't recreate the natural fetal environment entirely. But it might give Noah's lungs the time they need to develop further without the strain of mechanical ventilation."

7.2   The Artificial Placenta: A Step, Not a Leap

The artificial placenta was a technology born from decades of research, not as a complete solution but as a transitional step. Unlike an artificial womb, which could sustain a fetus in a fluid-filled environment with a functioning fetal circulation, the artificial placenta was designed for neonates who had already left the womb. By the time it was used, the natural advantages of fetal circulation—lower blood pressure, open shunts in the heart, and the remarkable oxygen efficiency of fetal hemoglobin—were already gone.

Instead, the artificial placenta connected directly to the baby's neonatal circulation through the umbilical vessels. Blood was drawn from the umbilical artery, passed through an oxygenator to remove carbon dioxide and add oxygen, and returned via *the umbilical vein. It functioned like ECMO but adapted for the smallest and most vulnerable patients.*

Dr. Moreau explained the procedure to Lina and her husband, Marco, with careful clarity. "The idea is to bypass Noah's lungs, allowing his blood to be oxygenated externally. He'll stay in his incubator, and you'll still be able to touch him. But there are trade-offs."

Marco leaned forward. "What kind of trade-offs?"

Dr. Moreau hesitated, choosing her words. "The artificial placenta doesn't recreate the natural environment of the womb. Noah will still be surrounded by tubes and wires. And while you'll be able to touch him, the setup is delicate, and any infection could be life-threatening."

7.3   A Difficult Choice

That night, Lina and Marco wrestled with their decision. The artificial placenta offered hope, but it was not the perfect solution they had imagined. Lina could not shake the thought of Noah's fragile skin, already marked by the interventions he had endured, being further exposed to the risks of infection.

"It feels like we're trying to bridge a gap that's too wide," she said, her voice breaking. "He's so tiny. Is this really what's best for him?"

Marco took her hand. "It's not perfect, but what if it's the only chance we have?"

They thought about the trade-offs: the opportunity to maintain some physical connection with Noah versus *the potential strain of being tethered to machines at such a vulnerable stage. Ultimately, they decided to proceed, hoping the artificial placenta could buy Noah the time his lungs needed to develop.*

7.4   The Fragility of Progress

The procedure was delicate. The surgical team worked with precision, threading cannulas into Noah's umbilical artery and vein. Monitors tracked every fluctuation in his vital signs as the system began its work. Blood flowed through the oxygenator, bypassing his struggling lungs, and returned enriched with oxygen.

For Lina and Marco, the sight of their son, still tethered to tubes and wires, was both a relief and a heartache. The artificial placenta stabilized Noah's oxygen levels, but the incubator remained a stark, clinical environment.

They could touch him through the incubator's access ports, but every interaction had to be cautious, mindful of the risks. Lina felt conflicted. On the one hand, she cherished the moments when Noah's tiny fingers wrapped around hers. On the other, she could not escape the thought that this was not how it was supposed to be. The constant presence of machines and the fear of infection cast a shadow over their bonding.

7.5   A Question of Balance

The researchers behind the artificial placenta had been candid about its limitations. Unlike an artificial womb, which sought to recreate the natural environment of pregnancy, the artificial placenta was a compromise. It provided life-saving support but lacked the holistic benefits of the fetal environment.

Dr. Moreau explained this during one of her check-ins with Lina and Marco. "The artificial placenta is a step forward, but it's not a perfect replacement for the womb. Without fetal hemoglobin and fetal circulation, we lose some of the natural advantages. And while you can touch Noah, we're constantly balancing that with the risk of infection."

Lina sighed. "Do you think this will ever feel … natural?"

Dr. Moreau smiled gently. "Natural? Maybe not. But it's a bridge. And bridges aren't where we stay—they're how we get to where we need to go."

7.6   A Fragile Hope

Over the next week, Noah's condition stabilized. The artificial placenta gave his lungs the rest they desperately needed, and the medical team began to see signs of improvement. Yet, the road ahead was still uncertain.

For Lina and Marco, the experience was bittersweet. They were grateful for the technology that had given their son a chance, but they could not help but wonder: Was this truly the best way forward? Could a more natural solution—like the artificial wombs they had read about—offer a better outcome in the future?

As they sat by Noah's incubator, watching his tiny chest rise and fall with increasing strength, Lina whispered, "You're so strong, little one. We're going to get through this together."

And in that moment, amid the tubes and monitors, they found a fragile hope— one that carried them through the uncertainty of today and into the possibilities of tomorrow.

7.7   Introduction

Over the past decade, the field of neonatal care has seen significant advancements with the development of two groundbreaking technologies: the artificial placenta (AP) and the artificial womb (AW). These technologies aim to improve the outcomes for extremely premature infants, those born before 28 weeks of gestation, by providing an environment that supports their development more effectively than current methods (Fig. 7.1).

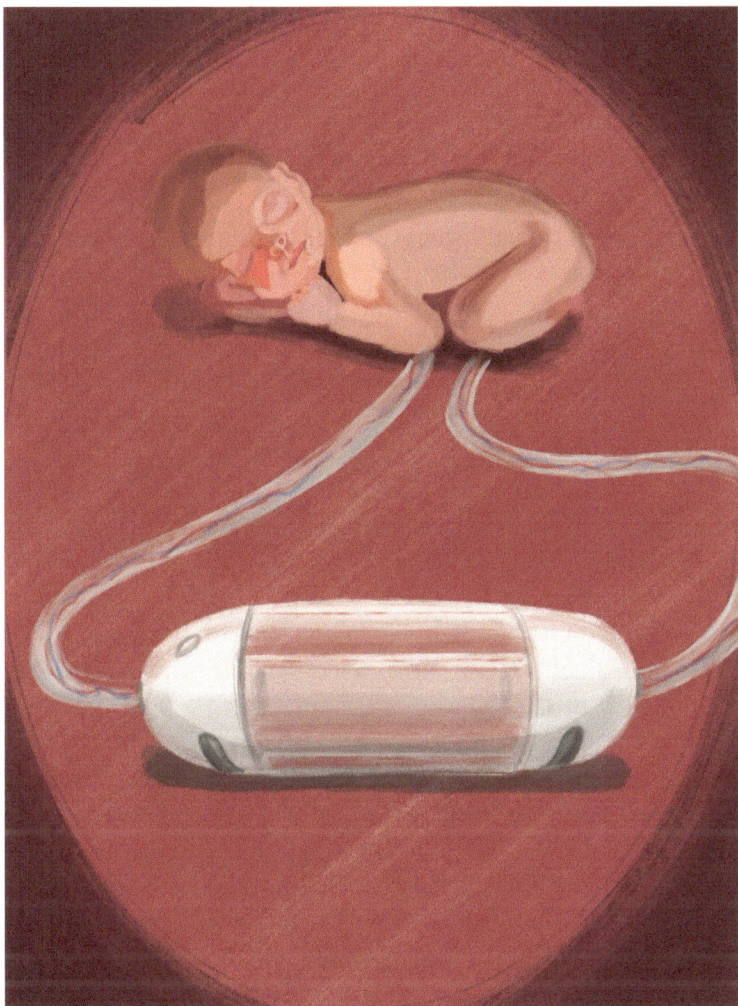

Fig. 7.1 Supporting the premature infant with oxygen and nutrients via an artificial placenta. This better reflects the dual function of gas exchange and nutritional support

7.8 The Challenges of Extreme Prematurity

For parents of extremely premature infants, the birth of their child can be a time of immense anxiety and uncertainty. These infants, classified as extremely low gestational age newborns (ELGANs), are born with severely underdeveloped organs. Traditional treatments, such as mechanical ventilation, while essential, often come with risks including lung damage and increased susceptibility to infections. The emotional toll on families is profound, with parents facing high levels of stress, anxiety, and depression as they navigate the complexities of caring for a preterm infant with multiple health issues

7.9 Background on Preterm Birth

When babies are born significantly earlier than their due date, particularly before 28 weeks of gestation, they are considered extremely premature. At this early stage, their organs, especially the lungs, are not fully developed, which makes survival outside the womb challenging

Two critical medical advances have significantly improved the chances of survival for these extremely premature infants: antenatal steroid therapy and surfactant replacement therapy

7.10 Antenatal Steroid Therapy

Antenatal steroid therapy involves giving steroids to the mother before delivery if there is a risk of preterm birth. These steroids help accelerate the development of the baby's lungs and other vital organs. Steroids stimulate the production of surfactant and other proteins essential for lung development, helping to prepare the lungs for breathing after birth. The steroids help reduce the risk of several complications associated with preterm birth, such as respiratory distress syndrome (RDS). By speeding up lung development, antenatal steroids have been a game changer, allowing babies born as early as 24 weeks to have a better chance of breathing on their own with medical assistance

7.11 Surfactant Replacement Therapy

Surfactant replacement therapy involves administering surfactant to the baby after birth. Surfactant is a substance that is naturally produced in the lungs and is essential for keeping the tiny air sacs (alveoli) open, allowing the baby to breathe properly. Surfactant reduces surface tension within the lungs, preventing the alveoli from collapsing. In premature infants, the lungs may not produce enough surfactant, leading to breathing difficulties and RDS. By giving surfactant therapy, doctors can help these infants breathe more easily. Surfactant replacement therapy has dramatically reduced the mortality rate and the severity of lung disease in premature infants. It has become a standard treatment for babies born with underdeveloped lungs

7.12 The Crucial Phase: 22–24 Weeks

The period between 22 and 24 weeks of gestation is a critical time for lung development, as the lungs begin to transition from the canalicular stage to the saccular stage. During the canalicular stage, the basic structures of the lungs form, but they do not yet support efficient gas exchange. The saccular stage marks the onset of alveoli development, the tiny air sacs where gas exchange occurs, and this is when the lungs begin to produce surfactant, becoming more capable of supporting breathing. By using antenatal steroid therapy and surfactant replacement, doctors can support and accelerate this crucial developmental phase, significantly improving the survival chances and overall health outcomes for extremely premature infants

7.13 Conclusion

The introduction of these therapies has been transformative in neonatal care. They have pushed the boundaries of viability, allowing babies born as early as 22–24 weeks to survive and thrive. These treatments are now standard practice in managing preterm births, providing critical support to the tiniest and most vulnerable patients

Despite these advancements, the lungs of babies born this early are still very immature. Current treatments, like positive pressure ventilation, help these infants breathe, but their lungs are not fully ready for the task. This can cause damage because their delicate lungs are exposed to mechanical stress and inflammation

7.14 The Artificial Placenta

Given these challenges, researchers have been looking for alternative ways to help these tiny infants breathe. One promising method is extracorporeal life support (ECLS), which has been around for over 50 years. ECLS involves taking over the job of the lungs and heart by circulating the blood outside the body to remove carbon dioxide and add oxygen. While ECMO has proven effective in older children and adults, it is not commonly used for very premature babies due to their fragile blood vessels and underdeveloped organs, which make the procedure too risky despite its potential benefits. ECMO mimics the function of the placenta during pregnancy by providing oxygen to the baby's blood and removing carbon dioxide, a key waste product. An artificial placenta could replicate this support for premature infants by delivering oxygen, aiding lung development, maintaining stable blood circulation, and bypassing the immature lungs, reducing the need for invasive ventilation

Fetal hemoglobin, the oxygen-carrying protein in a fetus's blood, is highly efficient even at low oxygen levels, making it particularly well suited for use with ECLS. Additionally, the umbilical vessels provide a safe and less invasive access point to connect the baby to the ECLS machine, minimizing trauma during the procedure. These unique features position ECLS—and particularly the development of an artificial placenta—as a promising solution to the respiratory challenges faced by extremely premature infants. As research progresses, the focus is on refining these technologies to offer better support and improve health outcomes for these vulnerable babies. The hope is that by mimicking the natural functions of the placenta, an artificial system could deliver oxygen, support lung development, and maintain stable blood circulation, all while reducing the need for invasive ventilation techniques. This innovation could revolutionize neonatal care, offering new hope to families and transforming the way healthcare providers manage premature birth

7.15 Milestones in the Development of the Artificial Placenta

The development of the artificial placenta is a story of remarkable innovation and determination, driven by the goal of improving survival rates for extremely premature infants. This journey began over half a century ago and has seen numerous advancements that have gradually brought us closer to a viable solution

7.16 Early Beginnings

The idea of using a heart–lung machine to support premature babies with respiratory distress emerged in the early 1960s. Callaghan and his team were pioneers in this field, conducting animal experiments to test the concept. In 1961, they used a Davol pump and a Pemco rotating disk oxygenator to create an early version of an artificial placenta. They connected the machine to both the femoral and jugular veins of the animals, directing the blood back into the heart. By 1962, Callaghan reported that this setup could keep dogs alive for an hour

7.17 Technological Advancements

Over the next decade, significant improvements in oxygenators and pumps made the artificial placenta more sophisticated and closer to its natural counterpart. Researchers began to use the umbilical vessels for connecting the machine, which provided a more natural route for blood flow. They also introduced parenteral nutrition, allowing the delivery of vital nutrients directly into the bloodstream. In 1969, Zapol and his team achieved a major milestone by keeping fetal lambs alive for more than two days using a silicone membrane oxygenator. This was a significant improvement, demonstrating that prolonged support was possible with better technology

7.18 Extending Survival

The late 1980s to the late 1990s saw further refinements in the artificial placenta, thanks to the work of researchers like Kuwabara and Unno. They managed to extend the survival time on ECLS to over three weeks. However, they faced challenges such as liver tissue damage due to the extra blood volume handled by the pump. They overcame this by introducing automated flow monitoring and control systems, which regulated the blood flow more precisely. Additional innovations included the use of a dialyzer and precise gas monitoring, which not only extended the survival time but also increased the system's complexity

7.19 Pumpless Circuits and Modern Developments

A significant breakthrough came in 1992 when Awad and his colleagues used a pumpless circuit for the first time as an artificial placenta. This system relied on the natural pumping action of the heart, reducing the need for complex machinery. They tested two commercially available oxygenators and found one that worked well for their lamb model, keeping the animals alive for up to six hours

In 1998, Dr. Sakata's team introduced a pulsatile centrifugal pump, which provided life support for up to 234 hours. While the survival time on pumpless ECLS systems was shorter than on more complex pump-driven systems, the simplicity and potential for less invasive application made it a focus of ongoing research

In 2009, Dr. Reoma and his team advanced the field further by using the Ann Arbor MC3 Oxygenator in a pumpless ECLS setup. They submerged lambs in artificial amniotic fluid and studied how the fetal circulation adapted to the ECLS system. They found that fetal blood flow patterns remained stable, although they noted a gradual decline in arterial blood pressure, limiting the duration of their experiments to around four hours

7.20 How the Artificial Placenta Works

The AP system connects to the infant's umbilical vessels, allowing blood to flow through an oxygenator where it is enriched with oxygen and cleared of carbon dioxide before being returned to the infant. This process bypasses the need for the infant to breathe air, which is vital for their delicate, underdeveloped lungs. Instead of air, the lungs are maintained in a fluid-filled state, supported by perfluorocarbon, a unique liquid with properties that help stabilize lung pressure and development

7.21 The Use of Perfluorocarbon

Perfluorocarbon plays a role in the context of advanced neonatal care due to its ability to carry oxygen and carbon dioxide efficiently. In some experimental setups, perfluorocarbons have been used to fill the lungs to help support their development without the risks associated with air ventilation. This substance helps to keep the alveoli open and reduces surface tension, promoting better gas exchange and lung growth. However, it is important to clarify that in the current implementation of the artificial placenta, the focus is primarily on the use of blood oxygenation through an extracorporeal circuit, and not necessarily on the use of perfluorocarbon within the lungs

The development of the artificial placenta at the University of Michigan has been a journey marked by significant challenges and remarkable innovations. Initially, researchers began with a system that did not use a pump. This early version of the artificial placenta relied on a transumbilical arterial–venous extracorporeal life support system, where blood was drained from the umbilical artery and returned via the umbilical vein in a fluid-filled environment. In these early experiments, five out of seven premature lambs survived for the four-hour study period, but all the animals eventually experienced a decline in cardiac function. The cause was identified as spasms in the umbilical artery, which led to reduced blood flow, low blood pressure, and insufficient oxygen levels

Recognizing the need to address this issue, the researchers transitioned to a veno-venous ECLS mode of support. In this improved system, blood is infused through the umbilical vein and drained from the jugular vein. The addition of a pump to this setup helped maintain a steady flow of blood, ensuring stable hemodynamics and gas exchange. By running the circuit parallel to the fetal circulation, rather than in series, this approach allowed the heart to pump against a more natural physiological load, reducing resistance and cardiac strain

7.22 The Role of Fluid-Filled Lungs

A crucial aspect of the artificial placenta's design is maintaining the lungs in a fluid-filled state, similar to the natural environment within the womb. Initially, researchers tried submerging the fetus completely in artificial amniotic fluid. However, this method led to fluid infections, prompting the need for an alternative approach. The solution involved intubating the fetus and filling the lungs with perfluorocarbons. Perfluorocarbons are unique liquids capable of carrying large amounts of oxygen and carbon dioxide, mimicking the properties of natural amniotic fluid. This method maintains appropriate pressure within the lungs and allows for fetal breathing movements, promoting normal lung development. Maintaining fluid-filled lungs through intubation and perfluorocarbons offers several advantages. It allows the infant to remain in a standard neonatal intensive care unit (NICU) incubator, facilitating normal nursing care, family bonding, and emergency access. This setup also simplifies the transition to air breathing. When the infant is ready, mechanical ventilation can be introduced, potentially using partial liquid ventilation as a bridge to full air breathing. This method ensures a smoother and safer transition from the artificial placenta to natural breathing

7.23 Successful Outcomes and Future Prospects

The veno-venous ECLS configuration with a pumping system has shown promising results in stabilizing blood flow and oxygenation in numerous studies. This system has even been tested as a rescue therapy for premature lambs that failed conventional mechanical ventilation, successfully reinitiating and maintaining fetal circulation

In the quest to improve the care of extremely premature infants, researchers in Aachen have been developing innovative technologies like the NeonatOx, a pumpless assist device. Unlike previous systems that relied heavily on pumps to fully replace the infant's lung function, the NeonatOx is designed to work alongside the baby's natural breathing. The NeonatOx is intended to be used as an assist device rather than a full substitute for lung function. This means it helps with breathing but does not completely take over the job. To make this possible, researchers have miniaturized the oxygenator, creating a custom device with a very small circuit volume of only 20 milliliters. For a model organism weighing around 1 kilogram, this is less than a quarter of its total blood volume

7.24 Benefits of Miniaturization

Miniaturizing the device brings several key advantages. Smaller, passively driven systems are less complex and easier to manage. They also pose fewer risks to the infant, such as blood damage, and are more portable. Additionally, because these systems have a lower filling volume, they reduce the need for blood transfusions. This is particularly important because blood transfusions can dilute fetal hemoglobin, increase inflammation, and have been linked to higher mortality rates in newborns

By minimizing the surface area of the device, the risk of blood clotting and inflammation is also reduced, making the device safer for long-term use

7.25 Nutrition of the Fetus

To ensure that a fetus can grow and thrive, delivering the right combination of nutrients is essential. The researchers have devised a highly controlled method of intravenous nutrition that provides the developing fetus with everything it needs to grow, mimicking the nutrient delivery provided by the mother in a natural pregnancy. A specialized intravenous solution is administered to the fetus. This solution is designed to provide a delicate balance of essential nutrients, ensuring proper growth and development. At the heart of the nutrient mixture is glucose, which comprises 10% of the solution. Glucose acts as a key energy source, powering the fetus's cellular activities and supporting its metabolic needs. Alongside glucose, the solution contains amino acids. These amino acids are crucial for the development of fetal tissues, particularly muscles and organs, as they serve as the building blocks for protein synthesis. Fats are also included, though in small amounts. These fats are essential for brain development and serve as an additional energy reserve for the fetus.

Vitamins and minerals round out the nutrient mix. A fraction of a multivitamin dose is administered daily to provide essential vitamins needed for cellular function and development. Additionally, a micronutrient solution, containing trace elements such as iron and zinc, is included to ensure that the fetus receives the necessary compounds for healthy growth. This intravenous nutrition delivers approximately 75 kilocalories per kilogram of fetal weight each day, providing just the right amount to support continued development in the artificial environment. By meticulously fine-tuning this delicate nutritional balance, the fetus receives the essential resources needed to grow as it would in the womb

7.26 Overcoming Natural Challenges

One challenge with an assist device rather than a full substitute for lung function is that it creates a unique circulatory situation that does not naturally occur. Normally, nature avoids having both the lungs and the placenta or an artificial equivalent working in parallel for gas exchange. Instead, there is an abrupt transition from fetal to adult circulation after birth

The artificial placenta is an exciting area of research that holds potential to transform neonatal care, but it is still in the experimental stages and far from ready for clinical use. While early studies suggest that it could provide a more natural and supportive environment for extremely premature infants, there are significant challenges that remain. These include ensuring long-term functionality, preventing complications such as infection or blood clotting, and addressing the technical difficulties of connecting the placenta to the baby's fragile blood vessels. Moreover, the artificial placenta's full impact on long-term health outcomes is still unknown, and it will take years of further research and clinical trials before it can be safely integrated into neonatal care. While the technology offers promise, it is important to temper expectations and acknowledge that many hurdles must be overcome before it becomes a reliable solution for preterm infant

8

The Artificial Womb: State of the Art

8.1 Bridging Two Worlds: An Obstetrician's Perspective

Dr. Beatrice Gouw stood at the edge of the NICU, her hands resting on the smooth surface of a transparent incubator. Inside, a tiny infant born at just 24 weeks fought for survival. The soft beeping of monitors punctuated the silence, each sound a stark reminder of the fragility of extreme prematurity. The baby's lungs, barely functional, strained against the ventilator's rhythmic support—a fragile line between life and loss.

As an obstetrician specializing in high-risk pregnancies, Dr. Gouw had spent her career balancing science, care, and hope. She had seen the miraculous resilience of preterm infants and the heartbreaking reality of those for whom the odds were too steep. The hardest cases, the ones that haunted her most, were the 24-week deliveries: babies brought into the world too soon, their tiny bodies unprepared for life outside the womb.

Her passion for improving outcomes in these cases was what drew her to artificial placenta technology. "It's not just about extending survival," she often said to her colleagues. "It's about creating the conditions for these babies to grow and develop as if they'd never left the womb. That's how we give them a real chance."

© The Author(s), under exclusive license to Springer Nature Switzerland AG 2025
G. Oei, *The Artificial Womb*, Copernicus Books,
https://doi.org/10.1007/978-3-031-85905-2_8

8.2   A Vision for Care Beyond Crisis

Dr. Gouw dreamed of a future where obstetricians could offer more than just emergency interventions. She envisioned a world where, after a premature birth, a seamless transfer to an artificial womb could preserve the baby's delicate physiology. In this ideal system, the infant's lungs wouldn't need to bear the burden of premature air exposure. Instead, oxygen would be delivered directly through the umbilical cord, mimicking the natural functions of the placenta.

Her vision was deeply personal. She had delivered hundreds of babies at the brink of viability, witnessed the anguish of parents unable to hold their newborns, and seen the long-term consequences of current neonatal practices. She knew that maintaining a fetal-like state outside the womb could mean the difference between a future marked by chronic illness and one full of potential.

However, she also grappled with the sacrifices this technology would require. Parents would no longer be able to cradle their newborns during those early, critical months. While touch was a cherished form of bonding, Dr. Gouw believed that for the baby, the artificial womb's cocooning environment was closer to nature than a NICU filled with tubes and alarms.

"But we must create new ways for parents to connect," she thought. "Touch might be limited, but their voices, their presence—those can still build the bond."

8.3   The Challenge of Natural Births

One of the hurdles Dr. Gouw felt strongly about was ensuring that artificial womb technology wouldn't inadvertently medicalize childbirth further. Most preterm infants delivered at 24 weeks or earlier were born via *cesarean section, as vaginal deliveries were deemed too risky. However, she believed that innovation should adapt to natural processes, not override them.*

Together with engineers and neonatal specialists, she had been working on a transfer system that could accommodate both cesarean and vaginal births. The idea was revolutionary: a fetus born prematurely could be gently captured in a sterile, fluid-filled transfer bag and seamlessly placed into an artificial womb without any invasive procedures or medication.

"Natural vaginal births must remain an option," she insisted in meetings. "If we make cesarean sections the default, we risk losing the essence of what childbirth is meant to be."

Dr. Gouw also recognized that any new technology must be both practical and sustainable. In an era of increasing healthcare costs, she knew that artificial womb systems would only succeed if they reduced the burden on hospitals rather than adding to it.

Her vision included self-correcting artificial wombs monitored remotely by technical physicians, allowing one clinician to oversee several cases simultaneously. This efficiency could not only lower costs but also free up medical staff to provide emotional support for families—a critical but often overlooked aspect of neonatal care.

Her goal was clear: the artificial womb should not be a luxury reserved for well-funded hospitals. It had to be accessible to all, including facilities in low-resource settings.

That evening, as Dr. Gouw prepared for another high-risk delivery, she paused by the NICU's glass doors. Inside, rows of tiny lives lay connected to machines—a reflection of both human resilience and the challenges of neonatal care.

The potential of artificial placenta technology filled her with hope, but she knew there was still much work to do. The technology had to evolve to preserve the dignity of childbirth, to ensure equity in access, and to provide a natural, nurturing environment for the most vulnerable.

"This isn't just about survival," she thought as she stepped into the delivery room. "It's about giving these children the future they deserve—one where they can thrive, grow, and live free from the scars of their earliest days."

As the birth unfolded, her resolve deepened. She would fight for this vision—for the mothers, for the babies, and for a world where being born too soon was no longer a life sentence but a beginning full of promise.

8.4   Introduction

The journey toward the development of an artificial womb has been marked by numerous pioneering experiments and significant advancements. Here, we explore the key researchers and their contributions during the foundational period of the 1960s and 1980s (Fig. 8.1).

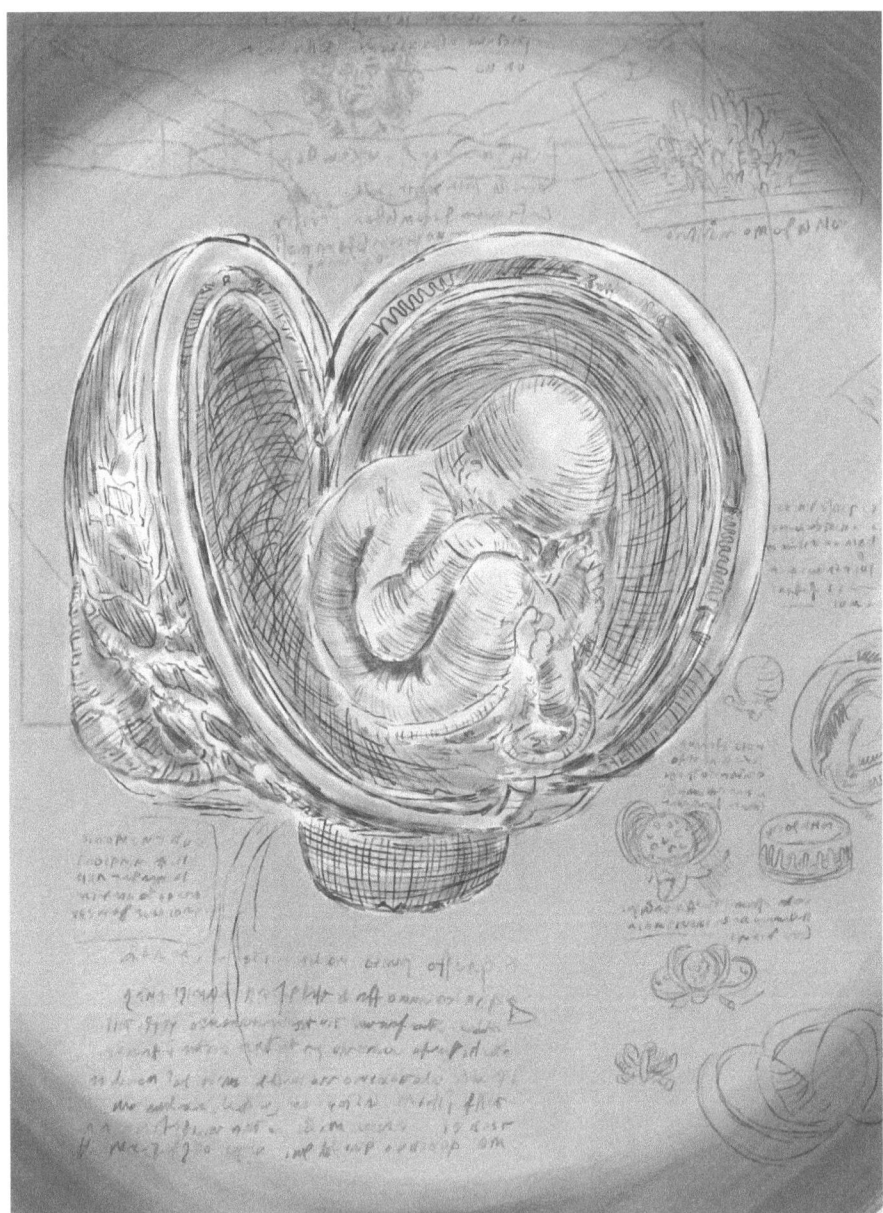

Fig. 8.1 Leonardo da Vinci's iconic sketches, including his detailed depiction of the uterus, juxtaposed with the Vitruvian Man, serve as a timeless exploration of human anatomy, now echoed in the quest to perfect the AquaWomb

8.5   Pioneering Researchers

The concept of the artificial womb, aimed at providing an optimal environment for prematurely born infants, has been the focus of scientific research for decades. The journey began with Emanuel Greenberg, who filed a patent in 1954 for an artificial uterus. Greenberg's design included a tank filled with amniotic fluid, an artificial kidney, two blood pumps, and a heating system, creating an environment to sustain a fetus and a placenta outside the womb. Although his invention never moved beyond the patent stage, it laid the groundwork for future innovations in neonatal care.

William Liley, a pioneering physiologist from New Zealand, made significant contributions to fetal physiology in the 1960s. He is best known for performing the first successful fetal transfusion in 1963, a groundbreaking procedure that treated Rh disease in utero. Liley's research into fetal development and intrauterine life contributed significantly to the understanding of the physiological needs of the fetus, which is critical for the development of artificial womb technology. Liley described the first treatment of Rh incompatibility with an intrauterine transfusion, an idea he conceived and executed based on his knowledge and experience. This treatment was later proven effective in randomized clinical trials. His pioneering work laid the groundwork for understanding how to manage and support a fetus inside the womb.

In Canada in 1961, John Callaghan and his team made significant strides with their experiments involving a heart-lung machine, similar to those used in cardiac surgeries. Their work focused on using extracorporeal life support (ECLS) to maintain gas exchange in fetal lambs. They employed a Davol pump and a Pemco rotating disk oxygenator to simulate the placental function. This early research demonstrated the potential of ECLS for sustaining fetuses but also highlighted the technical challenges involved. They successfully supported a preterm lamb for 21 hours in a device that provided oxygen to the lamb through its own umbilical cord, without it needing to breathe.

One of the early milestones in the quest to develop life-saving technologies for premature infants was the pioneering work of Robert Bartlett, a surgeon at the University of Michigan. During the 1970s and 1980s, Bartlett played a crucial role in the development of extracorporeal membrane oxygenation (ECMO), a revolutionary technology designed to treat newborns suffering from severe respiratory or cardiac failure. ECMO functions by diverting blood from the body, oxygenating it externally, and then returning it, effectively allowing the lungs and heart to rest and recover.

Initially, ECMO proved highly effective in treating full-term neonates and older children. However, despite its promise, its application in extremely preterm infants faced significant challenges due to their delicate physiology, particularly the fragility of their blood vessels and immature organs. As a result, ECMO never became a standard treatment for preterm infants, but its success in replicating certain placental functions—such as oxygenating the blood without the need for lung activity—sparked interest in developing alternative fetal support systems.

Bartlett's work not only transformed neonatal care for critically ill newborns but also laid the conceptual groundwork for future innovations aimed at supporting the development of extremely premature infants. His vision and achievements continue to inspire ongoing research into artificial placenta and womb technologies, as scientists seek to bridge the gap between extreme prematurity and viability.

The late 1970s and early 1980s saw Yoshinori Kuwabara in Japan making significant contributions. Kuwabara's experiments with goat fetuses were groundbreaking. He managed to maintain fetal goats in an artificial womb environment for several weeks. His work was notable for its focus on creating a liquid-filled environment that closely mimicked the conditions inside the womb. Kuwabara's presentations, such as the one at the FIGO World Congress in 1994, highlighted both the potential and the challenges of artificial womb technology, particularly issues related to infection control and long-term viability.

Marc Keirse played a pivotal role in bridging fundamental research and clinical application, particularly in obstetrics. Like Liley, Keirse was among the first to translate new ideas into practice based on knowledge and experience, daring to implement them clinically. He was a pioneer in prostaglandin research, leading to significant advancements in inducing labor and managing preterm birth. Additionally, he broke ground in treating pregnant women with recurrent miscarriages due to systemic lupus erythematosus (SLE) using heparin, laying the foundation for anticoagulation therapy in high-risk pregnancies. Both Liley's and Keirse's innovative approaches were later validated through rigorous randomized clinical trials.

Keirse's work extended far beyond individual therapies. He was instrumental in developing systematic reviews in perinatology and played a key role in initiatives like the Oxford Database of Perinatal Trials, which evolved into the Cochrane Database—a cornerstone of evidence-based medicine. Alongside Ian Chalmers and Murray Enkin, Keirse co-edited the landmark book *Effective Care in Pregnancy and Childbirth*, elevating the standards of perinatal research and ensuring its integration into clinical practice.

A critical lesson from Keirse's work is the importance of hemostasis in managing complex perinatal conditions. This principle is especially relevant to the development of artificial womb technologies, where maintaining proper coagulation is vital to the system's success. The knowledge gained from treating conditions like antiphospholipid syndrome with heparin and aspirin provides a crucial framework. These therapies, proven effective in preventing clot formation and ensuring adequate blood flow, could play a significant role in achieving stable hemostasis within the artificial womb environment.

Keirse's dedication to evidence-based medicine not only advanced perinatal care but also established a model for testing and implementing innovative technologies. His legacy underscores the importance of combining rigorous scientific evaluation with clinical integration, setting a clear precedent for how the artificial womb should be assessed and adopted in medical practice.

8.6   Challenges and Learnings

Researchers faced several critical challenges in their quest to develop systems that could replicate the womb environment for a developing fetus. One of the most pressing issues was infection control. Maintaining a sterile environment was paramount, as even the smallest exposure to pathogens could have devastating consequences for the fetus. This proved to be a significant hurdle, requiring innovative approaches to both equipment design and procedural protocols. Another challenge was nutrient delivery. Ensuring that the fetus received adequate nutrition while attempting to replicate the complex functions of the placenta was far from simple. The placenta is an intricate organ that not only provides nutrients but also manages waste and regulates essential hormones. Mimicking these processes outside the womb introduced layers of complexity that early researchers struggled to address with the limited technology of the time. Perhaps the most difficult obstacle was oxygenation and gas exchange. Developing a system that could manage the exchange of oxygen and carbon dioxide without damaging the delicate fetal tissues was particularly challenging. The fetus's reliance on the placenta for oxygen in the womb is a finely tuned process, and early experiments grappled with creating an external system that could replicate this without causing harm. Despite these challenges, the experiments of the 1960s and 1970s laid the groundwork for future advancements. Although constrained by the limitations of the era's technology, they provided invaluable insights into the physiological needs of a developing fetus and highlighted the complexities involved in mimicking the womb environment. These early learnings paved the way for the technological breakthroughs that would follow in the decades to come.

The 1990s saw significant advancements in Extracorporeal Membrane Oxygenation (ECMO) technology, which provided a basis for developing more sophisticated artificial womb systems. ECMO is a life-support technique that oxygenates blood outside the body, which is critical for supporting the underdeveloped lungs of premature infants. Researchers began integrating ECMO with artificial womb concepts to improve fetal support systems.

The early 2000s brought renewed interest and technological progress in the field. Advances in materials science, biomedical engineering, and neonatal care provided new tools and techniques for developing artificial wombs. Researchers focused on creating biocompatible materials, improving nutrient delivery systems, and enhancing the control of environmental conditions within the artificial womb.

8.7   Hollow Fiber Technology in Artificial Placenta and Artificial Womb Systems

One of the key technological advancements that has enabled the development of artificial placenta and artificial womb systems is hollow fiber membrane technology. Originally developed for applications like extracorporeal membrane oxygenation and dialysis, this technology is now being adapted to replicate the essential functions of the placenta, offering a lifeline to extremely premature infants. The integration of hollow fiber membranes into these systems is critical for mimicking the physiological conditions that support fetal development in utero. Hollow fiber membranes are composed of thousands of tiny, tube-like fibers that allow for efficient gas and fluid exchange. In an artificial placenta or womb system, these fibers are arranged to facilitate the transfer of oxygen and carbon dioxide, just as the placenta does naturally. Blood from the fetus circulates through the hollow fibers, where oxygen is supplied and carbon dioxide is removed, mimicking the gas exchange that would normally occur across the placenta. What sets hollow fiber technology apart is its low resistance. In fetal circulation, it is crucial to avoid placing too much strain on the developing heart. Hollow fiber oxygenators allow blood to flow through them with minimal resistance, making it possible for the fetus's own heart to drive circulation without the need for mechanical pumps. This pumpless design is a significant advantage, as it reduces the risk of complications such as cardiac failure or vascular injury, which can arise when the heart must pump against high resistance. The hollow fibers are typically made from biocompatible materials that ensure the blood flows smoothly and safely through the system. The thin walls of the fibers and their porous nature enable efficient gas exchange, with oxygen diffusing into the blood and carbon dioxide diffusing out. This process closely mirrors the natural function of the placenta, where maternal blood supplies oxygen and removes waste products from the fetal bloodstream. The large surface area provided by the hollow fibers ensures that this exchange is both rapid and effective, even when dealing with the small, fragile blood vessels of a preterm infant. This is crucial in artificial womb technology, where maintaining proper oxygenation is essential for the growth and development of organs, particularly the lungs and brain, which are vulnerable in premature infants. One of the primary challenges in supporting fetal life outside the womb is maintaining circulatory stability. The fetus relies on low-resistance pathways to ensure that blood can flow easily among the heart, lungs, and other organs. Hollow fiber technology addresses this need by offering near-zero resistance to blood flow, making it possible for the system to operate without overwhelming the fetal cardiovascular system. This low-resistance feature is especially important in artificial placenta systems that aim to support extremely premature infants. By mimicking the low-pressure environment of the fetal circulation, hollow fiber membranes allow the infant's heart to continue pumping blood efficiently without the added burden of mechanical pressure. This reduces the risk of cardiac stress and improves overall circulatory stability, giving the fetus a better chance of survival and healthy development. As artificial placenta and womb technologies evolve, hollow fiber membranes are proving to be a critical component in bridging the gap between research and clinical use. Their ability to provide efficient gas exchange and maintain low resistance makes them an ideal solution for mimicking the natural conditions of fetal development. With ongoing research and collaboration between medical institutions and technological innovators, hollow fiber technology continues to push the boundaries of what is possible in fetal care. As artificial placenta systems move closer to clinical trials, this technology will be central to ensuring the survival and healthy development of extremely premature infants.

8.8   The Philadelphia Experiment

A landmark study was published in 2017 by researchers at the Children's Hospital of Philadelphia. Led by pediatric surgeon Alan Flake, the team developed a device called the "biobag," an artificial womb that successfully supported the development of fetal lambs for up to four weeks. The biobag mimicked the amniotic fluid environment and used an umbilical cord interface for nutrient and gas exchange. This study demonstrated significant progress in maintaining fetal health and development outside the uterus and sparked widespread interest and optimism about the future of artificial womb technology. They reported the development of a system that features a pumpless oxygenator circuit connected to a lamb fetus via an umbilical cord interface, maintained within a closed "amniotic fluid" environment that closely mimics the conditions of the womb. They demonstrated that fetal lambs, developmentally equivalent to extremely premature human infants, can be physiologically supported in this extra-uterine device for up to four weeks. The lambs maintained stable hemodynamics, normal blood gas and oxygenation parameters, and intact fetal circulation. With appropriate nutritional support, lambs on this system exhibited normal somatic growth, lung maturation, brain growth, and myelination. The concept of a pumpless circuit powered by the fetal heart is not new and has been the initial approach for many researchers. Advantages include simplicity, the absence of pump-induced hemolysis, and the potential for some autoregulation of blood flow. However, disadvantages include the risk of cardiac failure due to afterload imbalance if the circuit or oxygenator has supraphysiologic resistance, or high-output cardiac failure if the resistance is subphysiologic. Most attempts have been limited by subphysiologic circuit flows and rapid hemodynamic decompensation despite vasopressor support. To address the limitations of subphysiologic flow in pumpless systems, most researchers have added pumps to arteriovenous systems. Although many attempts were short-lived and culminated in circulatory failure, prolonged survival of up to 543 hours was achieved in two fetal goats. However, this required dialysis, continuous paralysis, and ultimately resulted in respiratory failure. Hollow fiber plate technology has enabled the development of near-zero-resistance oxygenators, facilitating the creation of a pumpless system. In contrast to earlier studies, the researchers in Philadelphia did not observe any cases of cardiac failure in lambs at a developmental stage equivalent to 105 days of gestation and beyond. Notably, a low level of resistance developed across the circuit when using umbilical vascular access, which is consistent with some degree of autoregulation of blood flow.

Intracranial hemorrhage is a major concern in premature infants, raising issues about the use of anticoagulation in extracorporeal support systems. In Philadelphia, they used substantially reduced heparin doses compared with conventional ECMO. They attributed this reduction to the decreased surface area of their circuit and the inclusion of a heparin-bound coating on all blood-contacting components. Additionally, evidence suggests that germinal matrix hemorrhage is related to positive pressure ventilation and inotrope use, indicating that physiologic support in an extracorporeal system without ventilation or pressors may reduce hemorrhage risk. A critical feature of their system is the closed fluid environment with continuous fluid exchange. This preserves fluid-filled lungs and the normal glottic resistance required for maintaining airway pressures and lung development. Additionally, a fluid environment maintains the protective barrier between the fetus and the outside world. Fetal swallowing of amniotic fluid helps maintain fluid homeostasis and may provide an additional nutritional route. Continuous fluid exchange removes waste, maintains sterility, and mirrors the natural turnover of amniotic fluid. They have not encountered any significant infections since developing the Biobag.

8.9   Usuda and Kemp's Work in Perth

Around three months after the successful experiments in Philadelphia, Haruo Usuda and Matt Kemp in Perth, Australia, published their own successful experiment with preterm lambs using the Ex-Vivo Uterine Environment (EVE) therapy. Their research focused on maintaining key physiological parameters and preventing infections, achieving a stable environment for fetal development for up to a week. This parallel success further validated the feasibility of artificial womb technology and highlighted its potential for clinical application.

8.10   Toronto's Hospital for Sick Children, Canada

Christoph Haller and Mike Seed at Toronto's Hospital for Sick Children have been advancing artificial womb technology, primarily using fetal pigs as models. The Toronto team developed a "biobag" similar to the one used in Philadelphia, which creates an environment mimicking the amniotic sac by providing synthetic amniotic fluid. This setup supports fetal pigs, chosen for their anatomical and physiological similarities to human infants. However, the process remains highly experimental. The Toronto team has faced significant challenges, such as blood clotting and maintaining stable circulation. Despite these obstacles, they have successfully sustained fetal pigs in the artificial womb for about a week. While this progress shows potential, much work is still needed before the technology can be applied to human infants. Issues like ensuring long-term survival and preventing complications remain unresolved. Collaborations with other research institutions are ongoing to refine the technology and bridge the gap between animal models and potential human applications.

8.11 Eindhoven University of Technology, the Netherlands

At the Eindhoven University of Technology, a research group led by Professor Frans van de Vosse and Professor Guid Oei is developing the perinatal life support (PLS) system. Unlike other groups that use animal models, the Eindhoven team utilizes life-like fetal manikins and advanced computer simulations to closely mimic human fetal development. Their synthetic amniotic fluid environment supports fetal cardiorespiratory physiology, while their simulation technology validates the system without the need for animal models. This approach is designed to ensure a smooth transition to potential human clinical trials. The team collaborates with multiple international institutions, including RWTH Aachen University, Politecnico di Milano, and Toronto's Hospital for Sick Children to enhance their technology and prepare for clinical applications.

8.12 Hybrid Simulation Models

The development of life-like simulation models based on MRI images of a 24-week-old fetus represents one of the most innovative advancements in this field. These models are equipped with a beating heart and functioning lungs, allowing researchers to conduct realistic simulations. By integrating real patient data through computer simulations, these models provide accurate feedback on vital signs, such as temperature and oxygen levels, to predict the outcome of experiments. This approach ensures that researchers can refine their techniques and protocols in a controlled environment before moving to clinical trials with human subjects.

8.13 Transfer from Mother to Artificial Womb

The research team from Eindhoven has made an advancement with the development of a transfer system that works for both cesarean sections and vaginal births. In this system, the fetus is gently captured, almost like a goldfish, through a specialized lock mechanism and placed into a biobag. From there, the newborn is safely transferred into the artificial womb for further development. What makes this innovation truly revolutionary is that it eliminates the need to administer medication to the fetus during the transfer, preserving its natural state. Additionally, it allows for the use of the artificial womb even after a natural vaginal birth, a significant breakthrough. Previously, cesarean sections would have been necessary to place the newborn in the artificial womb, making the process more invasive than needed. This new method opens the door for less invasive, more flexible applications of the artificial womb, enhancing its potential in neonatal care.

8.14   Key Advances in Fetal Support: A Summary of Innovations and Impacts

Innovations in medical technology have led to breakthroughs in supporting extremely premature infants outside of the womb. One of the most significant advances is the use of hollow fiber oxygenator technology, which was first applied in ECMO during the 1980s. This innovation dramatically improved safety by reducing blood trauma and the risk of air embolism. Hollow fiber oxygenators use a semipermeable membrane to facilitate gas exchange without direct contact between blood and gas, creating a more stable environment for delicate neonatal physiology. The low-resistance design of these oxygenators enables efficient oxygenation of the baby's blood without requiring mechanical pumping, mimicking the natural function of the placenta. This advancement has not only enhanced ECMO technology but also laid the groundwork for developing artificial placenta systems aimed at supporting extremely premature infants. This has paved the way for a pumpless system, meaning the baby's own heart is strong enough to circulate blood through the system without external assistance. In previous systems, where pumps were needed to move blood, the added pressure often placed extra strain on the baby's heart, sometimes leading to cardiac failure as the heart struggled to keep up. However, in recent experiments with lambs that are developmentally similar to human fetuses at about 24 weeks of gestation, no such heart problems were observed. This is a critical improvement, as it shows that the system's low resistance design allows the heart to function naturally and safely. The use of umbilical vascular access, where blood enters and leaves through the umbilical cord, adds another layer of safety. It keeps the circuit's resistance low, meaning that blood can flow smoothly, and the baby's heart can keep pace without extra stress.

Additionally, the body's natural autoregulatory mechanisms, which help control and adjust blood flow, appear to still function in this setup. This is important because it suggests that the infants' body is able to adapt to the system in ways that keep blood pressure and flow at safe levels. This is particularly relevant for the brain, where sudden changes in pressure can lead to dangerous complications like intracranial hemorrhage, or bleeding in the brain. Brain bleeding, particularly in the form of germinal matrix hemorrhage, is a serious concern for premature babies, especially those born very early. This type of bleeding often occurs because the blood vessels in the brain are still very fragile and can be damaged by sudden increases in blood pressure or other stresses. Traditionally, premature infants who require mechanical ventilation and medications like inotropes—drugs that increase heart function—are at higher risk of this condition because both treatments can cause fluctuations in blood pressure and blood flow. One of the key advantages of an extracorporeal system is that it avoids these risks by eliminating the need for mechanical ventilation and inotropic drugs. Instead of forcing air into the baby's lungs, which increases pressure and can harm delicate tissues, the system keeps the lungs fluid-filled—just as they are inside the womb. This fluid environment maintains the fetus' natural lung development and helps preserve the gentle pressures needed for healthy growth. The system also avoids the use of inotropes because the fetus' heart is able to pump blood without extra help, reducing the risk of brain bleeds. In addition to controlling pressure, the system uses a reduced dose of heparin, a blood-thinning medication often used in systems like ECMO to prevent blood clots. Blood clots are a concern in any system where blood flows through tubes outside the body, but higher doses of blood thinners can also increase the risk of bleeding, including in the brain. To reduce these risks, the system uses heparin-coated components, meaning the surfaces that come into contact with blood help prevent clotting on their own. This allows for much lower doses of heparin to be used, which significantly reduces the risk of brain hemorrhages or other bleeding complications.

A crucial part of this system is its ability to mimic the natural fluid-filled environment of the womb. In the womb, a baby is surrounded by amniotic fluid, which not only cushions the baby but also plays a vital role in lung development. By keeping the baby's lungs filled with fluid, the system supports the natural development of the lungs without introducing air too early, which can lead to lung damage or conditions like bronchopulmonary dysplasia. The system also continuously exchanges fluid, which helps to maintain a sterile environment and mimics the way amniotic fluid is constantly renewed inside the womb. This fluid-filled environment also provides other benefits. For example, the fetus naturally swallows amniotic fluid during development, which is thought to help maintain fluid balance and may even provide some nutrients. By maintaining this process, the system supports the baby's normal development and growth. In addition, the continuous fluid exchange helps remove waste products, much like the placenta would in the womb, and ensures that the environment remains clean and sterile. Since this is a closed system, it also acts as a protective barrier, preventing the baby from being exposed to germs and infections from the outside world. Notably, since adopting this technology, no major infections have been reported, which highlights its effectiveness in maintaining a sterile environment. Despite these benefits, there are still some challenges to operating in this fluid-filled environment. For example, the fluid limits how much direct access caregivers have to the baby. In the case of emergencies, it might take longer to intervene, which presents some risks. However, the system can be designed with safety features to minimize these concerns. Caregivers can perform detailed ultrasound examinations that provide a clearer view of the baby's condition than traditional physical examinations. Additionally, the system includes access ports that allow caregivers to monitor the baby's blood flow, take blood samples, and provide nutritional support as needed, all without removing the baby from the protective fluid environment. There are also ports for meconium suction, which allow for the removal of waste if necessary. And, if an emergency arises, the system has been designed to allow rapid access for resuscitation. This means the fluid-filled "biobag" can be quickly opened so that medical teams can act without delay if the baby needs urgent care.

The combination of hollow fiber plate technology, a pumpless design, and a closed fluid environment holds the potential to revolutionize the care of extremely premature infants. By closely replicating the natural conditions of the womb, this system minimizes risks such as brain bleeds and infections, while also supporting critical lung development. As research and technological refinement progress, this approach could pave the way for a transformative new standard in neonatal care, offering a significantly improved pathway to survival for babies born far too early. Though challenges remain, this technology represents a significant step forward in neonatal care, providing a bridge between the womb and the outside world, where premature babies can continue to grow and develop safely.

8.15 Conclusion

The development of artificial womb technology has opened up exciting possibilities for improving neonatal care, particularly for extremely premature infants. However, it also presents significant challenges, particularly in the context of preventing brain hemorrhages and clotting disorders—common risks in premature babies due to the fragility of their blood vessels and low antithrombin levels. In the artificial womb, where an extracorporeal system like ECMO is employed, these risks are amplified. ECMO requires the use of heparin to prevent blood clotting, but this, in turn, increases the risk of hemorrhages, particularly in the brain. This is a significant problem when it comes to applying ECMO to premature infants, whose delicate systems make them highly susceptible to both clotting and bleeding complications.

A key challenge is the lack of an appropriate animal model to test these conditions. For example, while ECMO has been used in more mature infants and adults, it is rarely employed in extremely premature infants because of the increased risk of brain bleeds. Premature babies on mechanical ventilation face fluctuating blood pressure and heart function, which further exacerbates the risk of intracranial hemorrhages, particularly in the form of germinal matrix hemorrhages—a condition where the fragile vessels in the brain burst due to sudden pressure changes.

However, the artificial womb offers some potential advantages over traditional ECMO systems. One key difference lies in the maintenance of a persistent fetal circulation, meaning the blood flow is stabilized by shunts like the foramen ovale and ductus arteriosus, which are still open during fetal development. These shunts help maintain lower blood pressure and smoother circulation, reducing the risk of pressure fluctuations that could cause brain hemorrhages. Unlike ventilated neonates, who must adjust to breathing air, fetuses in an artificial womb remain in a fluid-filled environment, which stabilizes their lungs and circulation.

Moreover, the artificial womb uses a pumpless ECMO system, which minimizes turbulence in the blood flow. Turbulence can increase the likelihood of clot formation, so reducing this factor lowers the overall clotting risk. In this setup, the baby's own heart is responsible for circulating blood through the system, which helps maintain a steady, low-resistance flow without the need for external mechanical pumps.

In addition to these advantages, the fetus retains fetal hemoglobin, which allows it to efficiently carry oxygen at lower oxygen pressures, reducing the need for high oxygen levels that could otherwise exacerbate oxidative stress and damage fragile tissues. The lower pressures required in this system further contribute to minimizing the risk of brain bleeds, a crucial advantage over traditional ECMO systems used in neonates, where high pressures are a concern.

One of the most critical challenges, however, remains the lack of a reliable animal model to fully test these risks and benefits. While fetal lambs have been used in experimental models to approximate human fetal development at 24 weeks of gestation, these models do not perfectly predict human outcomes, especially regarding brain bleeding and clotting risks. Therefore, simulations and computational models are being developed to better understand how blood flow, pressure, and clotting interact in the artificial womb environment. These simulations allow researchers to model different scenarios and adjust parameters to optimize the safety and effectiveness of the artificial womb before moving on to human trials.

While these advancements show great potential, there remains a considerable journey ahead before the artificial womb can be safely and effectively integrated into clinical practice. Significant challenges must still be addressed, including optimizing the system for long-term use, ensuring the safety of the developing fetus, and refining the technology to prevent complications like blood clots and infections. Ongoing research and testing are crucial to overcoming these obstacles, and while progress is encouraging, widespread clinical application is still some distance away. More research is needed to address these technical and ethical challenges, and the development of better simulation models will be essential in guiding this research forward. Ultimately, the goal is to create a system that not only supports premature infants' survival but also minimizes the long-term risks of brain damage and other complications, offering a safer, more stable alternative to current neonatal intensive care methods.

As we continue to refine these technologies, it is critical to keep in mind the lessons learned from previous ECMO and fetal therapy efforts, balancing the promise of innovation with the need for caution and thorough validation. Through ongoing collaboration among patients, bioengineers, obstetricians, neonatologists, and ethicists, the artificial womb may one day revolutionize neonatal care and offer new hope to the most vulnerable infants and their families.

The state of the art in artificial placenta and womb technology is marked by significant advancements and innovative approaches. From the Biobag in Philadelphia to the sophisticated simulation models in Eindhoven, these technologies hold the potential to revolutionize neonatal care for extremely preterm infants.

The research groups are united by a shared goal and actively engage in international collaboration through conferences, joint studies, and shared publications. This global cooperation ensures that advancements and findings are disseminated widely, enhancing the collective understanding and development of artificial placenta and womb technologies. Such efforts are critical for moving closer to clinical applications that could revolutionize neonatal care, providing safer and more supportive environments for extremely preterm infants.

9

The Artificial Womb: Challenges and Solutions

9.1 A New Era in Neonatal Care

Dr. Emily Swan sat quietly in her small office, reviewing the details of her latest case. The soft murmur of the hospital around her was familiar, comforting even. As a young neonatologist, Emily was no stranger to the precarious balance of hope and uncertainty that defined her work. Every day brought new challenges, but today, as she prepared to meet a patient, she found herself reflecting on the evolving role of technology in her field.

That afternoon, Emily walked into the neonatal intensive care unit (NICU) to check on a baby born at 24 weeks gestation. The sterile hum of machines surrounded the tiny figure, and Emily's thoughts turned to the advances that were reshaping neonatal care. The artificial womb, once the realm of science fiction, was now a tangible reality in research labs. Although not yet ready for clinical application, its promise loomed large for families like those she served.

Later that evening, Emily attended a briefing on the artificial womb trials. The technology, still in its experimental stages, had shown immense promise. Unlike traditional NICU care, the artificial womb aimed to replicate the natural uterine environment, providing a fluid-filled chamber where a preterm infant could grow and develop. It offered an alternative to invasive ventilation and the many risks associated with traditional neonatal care.

Emily listened intently as the team discussed the latest breakthroughs. The transfer system, which allowed seamless transitions from the maternal womb to the

G. Oei, *The Artificial Womb*, Copernicus Books,
https://doi.org/10.1007/978-3-031-85905-2_9

artificial one, was particularly striking. It preserved the option for natural vaginal deliveries and ensured minimal disruption for the infant.

Her thoughts turned to the parents she worked with daily. How would this technology change their experience? Would it ease their fears or create new uncertainties? The team had introduced features like haptic feedback and audio systems to bridge the gap, allowing parents to feel and interact with their baby in ways previously unimaginable. "It's not perfect," Emily thought, "but it's a step closer to preserving the connection between parents and their child."

As Emily completed her rounds, she stopped to speak with a mother sitting by her baby's incubator. The woman's eyes, heavy with exhaustion, lit up as Emily approached. She asked questions about her baby's progress, and Emily explained each step with patience and care.

In that moment, Emily realized something profound. While the tools and techniques of neonatal care were changing, the essence of her work remained the same. It was not the machines or the methods that mattered most to the parents—it was the reassurance, the compassion, and the unwavering presence of someone who understood their fears and shared their hopes.

"For the parents, it's about feeling seen, supported, and understood," Emily reflected. No matter how advanced the technology became, her role as a guide and advocate for families would remain central. Holding their hands, answering their questions, and sharing in their journey—this was the heart of neonatal care.

As Emily returned to her office that night, she could not help but feel a renewed sense of purpose. The artificial womb represented a future filled with possibilities, but it was her connection to the families that grounded her work. The essence of neonatal care was not just about the survival of the infants; it was about the resilience of the parents, the strength of their love, and the dedication of those who walked alongside them.

Emily knew that while technology might change the tools she used, it would never replace the human touch at the core of her work. Whether in a bustling NICU or a world where artificial wombs became standard care, her role as a caregiver and guide would remain timeless.

9.2   Introduction

The development of artificial womb technology represents a profound leap in neonatal and perinatal care. This groundbreaking innovation offers the potential to bridge the gap between extreme prematurity and viability, providing a controlled environment where premature infants can mature in conditions that closely replicate the natural womb. While animal studies have demonstrated its feasibility, many challenges remain before this technology can be safely and effectively integrated into clinical practice. Addressing these challenges requires not only technical ingenuity but also ethical sensitivity and interdisciplinary collaboration (Fig. 9.1).

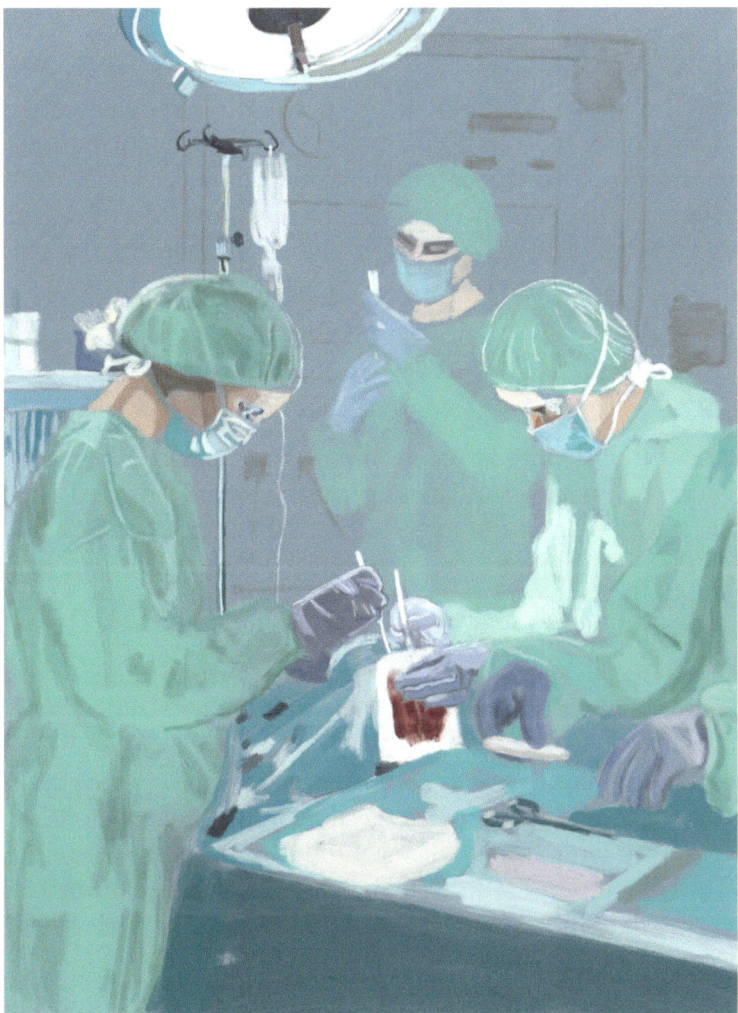

Fig. 9.1 Medical professionals in the process of transferring a fetus from the mother to an artificial womb, carefully connecting the umbilical cord to the artificial placenta—a crucial step in overcoming the challenges of bridging natural gestation with artificial support

9.3   Challenges and Solutions in Artificial Womb Technology: Ensuring a Safe Transition to the Biobag

Challenge Premature infants often face significant risks if they begin breathing before being placed in the artificial womb. The premature activation of the lungs can cause irreversible damage, increasing complications and reducing survival chances.

Solution The transfer from the maternal womb to the biobag must be meticulously controlled to maintain the fluid-filled state of the lungs, mirroring conditions in utero. Advanced imaging can guide this transition, ensuring that the fetus remains calm and stable. Gentle handling protocols, coupled with minimal use of sedatives or muscle relaxants, will further support a seamless transfer process.

9.4   Reducing the Need for Cesarean Sections

Challenge Cesarean sections, while lifesaving in many contexts, carry risks for the mother, including infection, hemorrhage, and longer recovery times. Additionally, when performed during extreme prematurity, a Cesarean section can leave a scar in the upper part of the uterus (the corpus), which increases the risk of complications in future pregnancies. These complications include a higher chance of the scar rupturing during labor and a condition called placenta previa, where the placenta covers the cervix and can cause severe bleeding. Such risks highlight the importance of minimizing unnecessary cesarean sections whenever possible.

Solution Developing a transfer system that accommodates both cesarean and vaginal births is essential. Innovative technologies, such as a specialized transfer bag that gently captures the fetus during vaginal delivery, can facilitate a smooth transition to the artificial womb. This approach prioritizes the health and safety of both the mother and the baby, making the process less invasive and more accessible.

9.5   Creating a Realistic Womb-like Environment

Challenge The artificial womb must replicate the complex biochemical, physical, and sensory environment of the natural womb to ensure proper fetal development. This includes temperature regulation, fluid dynamics, nutrient delivery, and even light and sound exposure. *Solution*: The biobag should incorporate advanced temperature control systems and a continuous supply of synthetic amniotic fluid enriched with essential hormones, growth factors, and nutrients. Sensors embedded in the system will monitor and adjust environmental parameters in real time, ensuring stability. Controlled lighting systems and sound transmission devices can mimic natural womb conditions, providing the fetus with familiar stimuli that support neurological and sensory development.

9.6 Strengthening Parental Bonding

Challenge One of the most significant concerns with artificial womb technology is the potential disruption of the emotional bond between parents and their baby. Traditional NICU settings often leave parents feeling disconnected due to physical and emotional barriers.

Balancing the Needs of the Baby and Parents In the natural womb, a fetus resides in a dark, enclosed environment, shielded from visual stimuli. This darkness is part of the natural development process, suggesting that a transparent biobag might not replicate the true conditions of the womb. While transparency could allow parents to see their baby, it is uncertain if this visibility benefits the baby or aligns with its developmental needs. A darker environment might better simulate the natural womb, fostering a sense of security for the fetus.

Parental Connection For parents, however, being able to see their baby might have psychological and emotional benefits. In traditional NICU settings, parents can see their baby through incubators, and this visual connection can be a source of reassurance. Research on fetal bonding during ultrasound examinations suggests that seeing the baby can enhance the parents' sense of connection, though concrete evidence on its long-term impact is limited.

Solutions The biobag could incorporate controlled transparency, allowing parents occasional visual access during specific moments, such as daily check-ins or supervised bonding sessions. This approach could balance the baby's need for a natural, darkened environment with the parents' desire to feel connected. Additionally, haptic feedback systems could allow parents to feel the baby's movements, replicating the sensation of kicks or shifts, which is a crucial part of prenatal bonding.

Building Connection beyond Sight Audio systems enabling parents to talk or sing to their baby could further strengthen emotional bonds. The sound of a parent's voice is known to comfort and stimulate fetal development. Real-time monitoring, video feeds, or occasional visual glimpses could also reassure parents about the baby's well-being without compromising the simulated womb environment.

A Balanced Approach Ultimately, the design of the artificial womb must prioritize the baby's developmental needs while providing parents with meaningful ways to connect. Just as in the NICU, where parents are encouraged to engage in skin-to-skin contact and other bonding activities, artificial womb technology should explore ways to preserve and enhance this connection in a manner that supports both the baby and the parents.

9.7 Managing Medical and Technical Complexities

Challenge Maintaining a sterile and stable environment for the fetus is a formidable challenge, as even minor disruptions can lead to infections or developmental complications. Additionally, issues like inflammation, clotting, and the complexity of cannulation must be addressed.

Solution Advanced materials with antimicrobial properties and robust sterility protocols will minimize infection risks. For inflammation and clotting, incorporating surface coatings that reduce reliance on anticoagulants like heparin can help maintain fetal health. Cannulation techniques must be refined, with flexible, biocompatible cannulas that ensure secure attachment and optimal blood flow.

9.8 Addressing Ethical and Legal Considerations

Challenge The use of artificial wombs raises profound ethical and legal questions, including the definition of fetal rights, the implications of extending viability limits, and the societal impact of such transformative technology.

Solution A comprehensive ethical framework must be developed, engaging bioethicists, legal experts, and diverse communities. Clear guidelines should define the legal status of a fetus in an artificial womb, covering parental rights, medical decision-making authority, and broader societal responsibilities.

Public education campaigns and dialogues will help demystify the technology and build trust.

9.9   Ensuring Accessibility and Usability for Low-Resource Settings

Challenge The potential for artificial womb technology to save lives hinges on its accessibility across diverse healthcare environments, particularly in low-resource settings where preterm birth rates are often highest. However, the approach to making this technology accessible in such environments requires careful consideration.

Solutions Balancing simplification and innovation of simplified designs may initially seem like the most practical solution for low-resource countries, with features like solar-powered systems reducing dependency on unreliable infrastructure. These designs could lower costs and make the technology more deployable. However, the critical shortage of highly trained medical personnel in these settings introduces another layer of complexity.

9.10   Leveraging Artificial Intelligence and Digital Twin Technology

Rather than purely simplifying the system, leveraging advanced technologies such as artificial intelligence (AI) and digital twin models could address personnel shortages by shifting from decision support to decision-making systems. Digital twins—a real-time virtual representation of the fetus within the artificial womb—could monitor, predict, and optimize care by simulating potential outcomes and suggesting adjustments. AI-driven decision-making could reduce the need for constant oversight by specialized clinicians, enabling one physician to oversee multiple systems simultaneously. This shift would ensure that the technology remains effective without requiring extensive medical expertise on-site.

9.11   Global Collaboration and Cost Efficiency

Collaborative global efforts are needed to develop these systems at scale, ensuring affordability through economies of scale. Public and private partnerships could fund the development and deployment of these advanced systems.

Moreover, local training programs could empower healthcare workers with the knowledge to operate and maintain the technology.

9.12 Striking the Right Balance

While simplified, solar-powered systems may serve as a stepping stone, integrating AI and digital twin technology could provide a more sustainable, long-term solution for low-resource environments. These advanced systems, when paired with targeted training, could enhance the accessibility and usability of artificial womb technology globally, ensuring that even the most vulnerable populations benefit from these lifesaving innovations.

9.13 Preparing for the First Human Trial

Challenge Conducting the first in-human trial is one of the most critical and delicate steps in the development of artificial womb technology. It requires meticulous planning and rigorous ethical oversight to ensure safety and efficacy.

Solution A phased, stepwise approach should guide the transition to human trials:

1. *Preclinical validation*: Extensive testing on animal models to refine protocols and identify potential risks.
2. *Simulations*: High-fidelity simulations using digital twin technology to model potential outcomes and refine procedures.
3. *Ethical review*: Comprehensive review by ethics boards to ensure transparency and public accountability.
4. *Training programs*: Developing detailed training protocols for medical teams, including contingency planning.
5. *Phased clinical trials*: Starting with a small, closely monitored trial population before scaling up based on outcomes.

9.14 Evaluating Long-Term Effects

Challenge The long-term physical, mental, and developmental impacts of artificial womb technology remain unknown, raising questions about its safety and efficacy overtime.

Solution Longitudinal studies must track children born through artificial womb systems, monitoring health outcomes over years and decades. These studies will provide invaluable data to refine the technology and address any unforeseen challenges.

9.15 Fostering Public Understanding and Acceptance

Challenge Misconceptions, fears, and ethical concerns about artificial womb technology can hinder its adoption and integration into healthcare systems.

Solution Transparent communication and public education initiatives are essential. Collaborating with media, community leaders, and advocates can help build a nuanced understanding of the technology's benefits and limitations, fostering informed discussions and societal acceptance.

9.16 Conclusion

The path to implementing artificial womb technology in clinical practice is complex, requiring interdisciplinary collaboration, rigorous ethical oversight, and a commitment to accessibility and equity. While significant challenges remain, the solutions outlined here offer a roadmap for navigating this transformative journey. By addressing each obstacle thoughtfully and systematically, artificial womb technology has the potential to redefine neonatal care, offering hope and a brighter future for countless families worldwide.

10

The Artificial Womb: Future Perspective

10.1 Leapfrogging into the Future: Artificial Womb Technology in Uganda

Dr. Kwoba, a visionary entrepreneur and founder of Ubuntu Birth Solutions, stood at the entrance of a bustling medical center in Kampala, Uganda. A young couple rushed past, their premature baby swaddled in a cloth, its fragile body struggling for breath. Scenes like this were at the heart of why Kwoba founded his company—to provide innovative solutions for the challenges facing maternal and neonatal care in Uganda. With a focus on sustainability and accessibility, Kwoba's team was pioneering the integration of artificial womb technology into the country's healthcare system.

As a leader deeply committed to addressing Uganda's healthcare challenges, Kwoba recognized the dire need for scalable, sustainable solutions in a country where neonatal mortality rates remained high. Uganda's healthcare system, like many in low-income countries, faced significant limitations: a shortage of highly trained medical staff, unreliable electricity, and limited access to advanced medical technologies.

"Our goal isn't just to introduce new technology," Kwoba explained. "It's to create solutions that work for Uganda—innovations that are affordable, durable, and tailored to our unique circumstances."

Ubuntu Birth Solutions focused on leveraging technology to address gaps in neonatal care, with the artificial womb as its flagship initiative. The company partnered with international universities, engineers, and local healthcare providers to co-create systems designed specifically for low-resource environments.

© The Author(s), under exclusive license to Springer Nature Switzerland AG 2025
G. Oei, *The Artificial Womb*, Copernicus Books,
https://doi.org/10.1007/978-3-031-85905-2_10

Kwoba's team turned potential barriers into opportunities by prioritizing simplicity and efficiency. Unlike traditional neonatal intensive care incubators, which required constant monitoring and highly trained staff, the artificial womb system was designed to be largely autonomous. Sensors and algorithms regulated oxygen levels, nutrient delivery, and temperature, minimizing the need for human intervention.

The use of solar-powered systems ensured that the technology could function in areas with intermittent electricity, while artificial intelligence (AI)-driven decision-making reduced the reliance on specialized personnel. "By integrating AI and digital twin technology," Kwoba noted, "we can make advanced neonatal care accessible even in the most remote clinics."

A cornerstone of Ubuntu Birth Solutions' success was its collaborative approach. Kwoba worked closely with local communities, parents, and healthcare providers to ensure that the technology met their needs. Focus groups revealed concerns about bonding, which led to the inclusion of features like real-time video feeds, audio connections, and haptic feedback systems that simulated the baby's movements.

"Parents play a crucial role in their baby's journey," Kwoba emphasized. "We designed the system to enhance that connection, not replace it."

The company also partnered with international institutions to incorporate cutting-edge technology, such as digital twin modeling. This allowed real-time simulation of the baby's development, enabling precise adjustments to the artificial womb environment and improving outcomes.

The transformative potential of the artificial womb became evident with its first use. A young couple arrived at one of Ubuntu's partner clinics when the mother unexpectedly went into labor at 26 weeks gestation. While 26 weeks marks the current limit of viability in Uganda, many babies born at this stage face significant risks of severe complications, including lifelong disabilities. This time, however, the couple's baby had access to a revolutionary option: the artificial womb.

Immediately after delivery, the baby was gently transferred into a specialized transfer bag, ensuring the lungs remained fluid-filled and protected from premature exposure to air. This critical step allowed for a smooth transition into the artificial womb, where the baby's development could continue under optimal conditions.

Inside the artificial womb, the system's controlled, fluid-filled environment supported the baby's lungs and other organs as they continued to grow and mature. The technology not only focused on survival but also prioritized reducing the risks of complications that often accompany extreme prematurity, such as brain injuries, respiratory problems, and developmental delays.

For the parents, the experience was transformative. Through the biobag's transparent window, they could observe their baby's tiny movements and hear its steady heartbeat, providing a sense of connection during a challenging time. Features like audio systems enabled the parents to speak and sing to their baby, fostering a bond even within this advanced technological environment.

By focusing not only on survival but on healthy survival without major disabilities, Ubuntu's artificial womb program represents a critical step forward in neonatal care in low-resource settings like Uganda, where the burden of prematurity remains high.

One of Ubuntu Birth Solutions' defining features was its commitment to sustainability. The company designed the artificial womb to be cost-effective, with locally sourced components and energy-efficient systems. Solar power and AI-driven automation reduced operational costs, making the technology accessible to clinics across Uganda, even in rural areas.

Kwoba's vision extended beyond Uganda. "We're creating a model that other low-resource countries can adapt," he explained. "This isn't just about Uganda—it's about reimagining neonatal care for the entire Global South."

While the program's success was inspiring, challenges remained. Ethical questions surrounding the artificial womb required careful consideration, and ensuring equitable access was an ongoing priority. Kwoba's team worked closely with policymakers and bioethicists to develop guidelines that balanced innovation with societal values.

"There's no one-size-fits-all solution," Kwoba acknowledged. "We need to keep refining the technology while addressing the cultural and ethical nuances of each community we serve."

The success of Ubuntu Birth Solutions in Uganda quickly garnered international attention. Delegations from Kenya, Tanzania, and Malawi visited to learn from the model, while global conferences highlighted Uganda's approach as a blueprint for integrating advanced medical technologies into low-resource settings.

For Kwoba, the greatest reward was seeing families reunited with healthy, thriving babies. "Every life saved is a testament to what's possible when innovation is driven by empathy and collaboration," he said.

Looking ahead, Kwoba envisions a world where no child is lost to prematurity. His team is already exploring ways to expand their work, from developing portable versions of the artificial womb to creating training programs for healthcare providers.

"The artificial womb is more than just a piece of technology," Kwoba reflected. "It's a symbol of hope—proof that even in the face of limited resources, we can find solutions that transform lives."

Through Ubuntu Birth Solutions, Kwoba is not only redefining neonatal care in Uganda but also inspiring a global shift in how healthcare innovation can meet the needs of the most vulnerable.

10.2 Introduction

The development of artificial womb technology holds the promise of transforming neonatal care and medical research, with potential to redefine the care of premature infants and accelerate scientific advancements (Fig. 10.1).

This chapter outlines the significant potential of artificial womb technology, emphasizing its benefits for medical research, clinical preparedness, and neonatal care efficiency. It also highlights the broader ethical, societal, global,

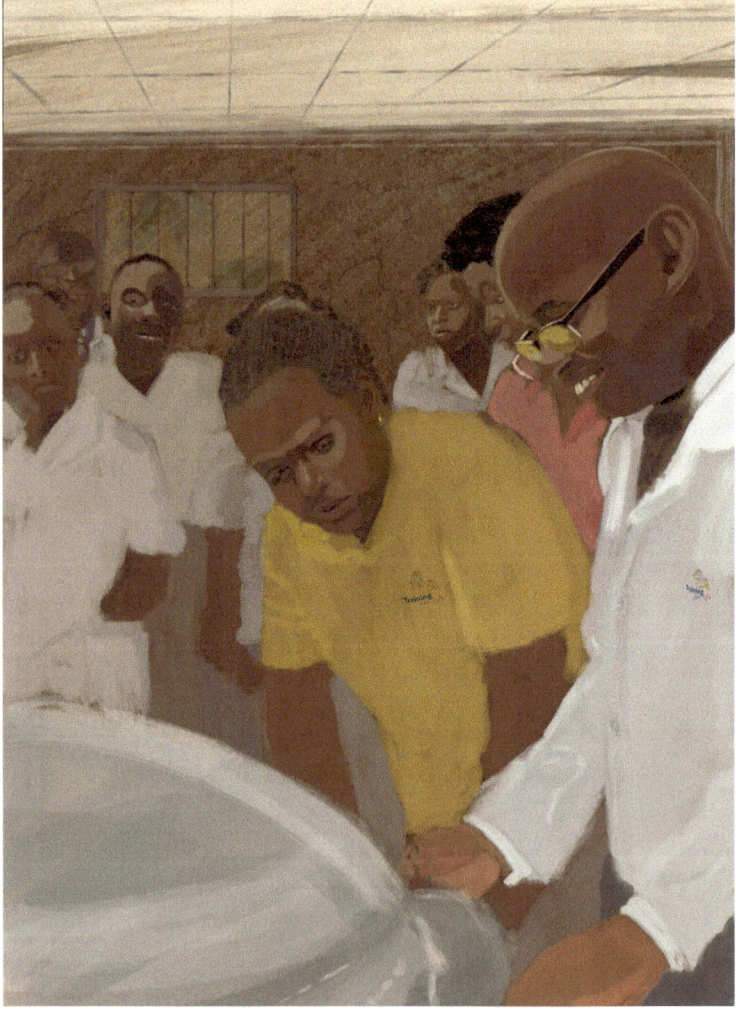

Fig. 10.1 Doctors in Uganda working with an artificial womb, showcasing the potential of new technologies to improve neonatal care and outcomes for premature infants in regions with limited healthcare resources

and economic considerations that must be addressed as this technology progresses. Though still in its developmental stages, artificial womb technology provides a glimpse into a future where premature infants can mature in an environment that closely mimics the natural womb, significantly improving survival rates and long-term health outcomes.

The development of artificial womb technology is set to revolutionize neonatal care and medical research, offering a transformative approach that promises to redefine standards and practices across a broad spectrum of clinical applications. This future perspective encompasses the creation of sophisticated simulation models, advanced sensor technology, and artificial intelligence (AI), all converging to provide an unprecedented platform for nurturing and studying extremely premature fetuses.

10.3 Advanced Simulation Models and Digital Twins

At the core of this technological breakthrough are highly advanced simulation models designed to replicate the physical and biological responses of extremely premature fetuses. These models, equipped with a comprehensive array of cutting-edge sensors, function as digital twins of real 24-week-old fetuses. This digital twin technology provides a precise and reliable means of understanding how a fetus at such a critical stage of development would respond to various medical interventions and environmental conditions.

The implications of this technology for medical research are profound. Traditionally, researchers have relied heavily on animal models to simulate human conditions. However, significant physiological differences between species often limit the applicability of these models. The digital twin technology employed in artificial wombs overcomes these limitations by offering a closer approximation to human physiology. This breakthrough ensures that research findings are more relevant and applicable to human health, bridging the gap between preclinical studies and human clinical trials.

10.4 Enhancing Medical Research and Clinical Preparedness

The ability to repeatedly practice and refine medical procedures using these simulation models before conducting actual human experiments marks a significant advancement in medical research. This approach ensures that medical teams are exceptionally well prepared, minimizing risks and enhancing the safety and efficacy of neonatal care procedures. Such thorough preparation is crucial for improving outcomes in premature infants, who are particularly vulnerable and require highly specialized care.

Furthermore, the integration of clinical decision support systems with these models represents a significant leap forward in medical technology. These systems leverage the power of artificial intelligence to combine physiological and mathematical models, autonomously managing critical parameters such as oxygen supply, nutrient delivery, and other vital functions. This integration creates a plug-and-play solution, where the system operates automatically once the umbilical cord is connected to the artificial placenta. Such autonomous operation significantly reduces the need for continuous human intervention, allowing a single medical engineer or technical physician to monitor and manage multiple systems simultaneously.

10.5 Addressing Nursing Shortages and Enhancing Care Efficiency

The efficiency of the artificial womb system is particularly crucial given the anticipated global shortage of nursing staff. Currently, the care of premature infants in incubators requires round-the-clock attention from dedicated nursing staff. This intensive care demand poses a significant challenge, especially in regions with limited healthcare resources. The artificial womb technology mitigates this issue by enabling more efficient use of medical personnel. A single technical physician can oversee the operation of several artificial wombs, ensuring that high-quality care is maintained despite staffing constraints.

This vision extends to the complete replacement of traditional incubators with artificial wombs, allowing fetuses to reach full maturity in a controlled, natural-feeling environment. This technology facilitates perfect bonding opportunities with parents, providing a better start for the child even before birth. By allowing the fetus to develop in conditions that closely mimic the natural womb, the artificial womb helps mitigate the long-term developmental delays often seen in late preterm infant delays that many never fully overcome.

10.6 Global Impact and Accessibility

The potential impact of artificial womb technology extends beyond high-resource settings. In low-income countries, where healthcare resources are often severely constrained, this technology could prove to be a game-changer.

In many of these regions, incubators often remain unused due to a lack of trained nursing staff. The artificial womb system, with its autonomous operation and minimal staffing requirements, can fill this critical gap, providing effective care for premature infants who might otherwise not survive.

In many low-income countries, particularly in Sub-Saharan Africa, technology has played a crucial role in overcoming traditional infrastructure limitations. This phenomenon, often referred to as "leapfrogging," allows nations to bypass certain stages of development and adopt newer, more advanced technologies directly. One striking example is the widespread use of mobile phones in regions where fixed landlines were never established on a large scale.

In much of Sub-Saharan Africa, the cost and complexity of installing landline telephone networks proved impractical. Instead of investing in outdated infrastructure, these countries embraced mobile technology, providing people in remote areas, who were once isolated, with access to communication via mobile phones. This shift has not only improved communication but also broadened access to information, healthcare, and education, particularly in rural communities.

Similarly, many people in low-income countries have leapfrogged traditional banking systems in favor of mobile payments. In Kenya, for instance, the mobile payment platform M-Pesa has become an integral part of the economy. This service allows individuals without bank accounts to transfer money, pay bills, and make purchases using their mobile phones. For many, particularly in rural areas, the smartphone has become their primary financial tool, facilitating access to a range of services from microloans to international transactions.

The concept of leapfrogging offers promising opportunities for introducing cutting-edge medical technologies, such as artificial placentas and artificial wombs, into low-income countries. Rather than investing in costly, labor-intensive neonatal care systems like traditional neonatal intensive care units (NICUs) with one-to-one care, these nations could potentially leap directly to more automated and efficient solutions. Technologies like the artificial womb could revolutionize the care of premature infants, enabling countries without extensive healthcare infrastructure to rapidly catch up with more advanced systems.

These innovations could have a profound impact by reducing the reliance on expensive and scarce healthcare staff while harnessing scalable technological solutions that require less human intervention. Just as mobile phones and mobile banking transformed entire regions, advanced medical technologies could improve neonatal care in areas that have historically been limited by infrastructure challenges.

This leap to new technologies presents not only a path forward for healthcare in low-income countries but also a means to reduce disparities in access to care. By overcoming technological barriers, these nations could benefit from the same innovations used in wealthier countries, but in a more cost-effective and accessible manner, thus narrowing the healthcare gap on a global scale.

The World Health Organization (WHO) has identified reducing neonatal mortality due to premature birth as a top global health priority. Premature birth is a leading cause of infant mortality worldwide, particularly in low-income countries. The WHO has set ambitious targets to decrease infant mortality rates significantly in the coming decades. The artificial womb technology is poised to play a pivotal role in achieving these targets offering a lifeline to countless infants and their families.

By providing a reliable and effective means of nurturing premature infants, artificial wombs can help reduce the incidence of neonatal mortality and morbidity. This technology not only saves lives but also improves the quality of life for survivors by reducing the risk of long-term health complications associated with premature birth. The ripple effects of such improvements extend to families and communities, fostering better health outcomes and economic stability.

10.7 Ethical and Economic Considerations

The development of artificial womb technology presents a groundbreaking opportunity to address critical ethical concerns in medical research while offering promising solutions for premature infants. By moving away from animal testing, this technology adheres to a forward-thinking approach that resonates with broader societal values regarding humane and ethical treatment of animals. Eliminating animal models not only alleviates ethical concerns but also enhances the relevance and applicability of research findings for human clinical use.

At present, no research groups are working on complete ectogenesis, the process of developing a fetus entirely outside the womb. However, several teams are advancing significantly in early embryo development, exploring how to support embryos outside the human body for a limited period. Before bridging the gap from early embryo development to artificial womb technology for premature infants, it is crucial to have an open and transparent ethical debate. This dialogue should involve scientists, ethicists, medical professionals, and the public, ensuring that the ethical implications of such a profound leap in reproductive science are thoroughly considered.

Public engagement, through platforms such as social media and films, plays a vital role in shaping this debate. These media can help demystify the technology, address concerns, and stimulate informed discussions on its future. Ethical co-creation ensures that the evolution of artificial womb technology aligns with societal values while advancing neonatal care.

10.8 Co-creation with Patients

Involving patients in the design process of innovative medical technologies, such as the artificial womb, is crucial for creating solutions that truly meet the needs of those who will be most affected. Parents who have experienced the emotional and medical challenges of extreme preterm birth have a unique understanding of what an artificial womb should offer, especially regarding aspects like safety and bonding. Their insights are invaluable, as they bring real-world perspectives that healthcare professionals and engineers might overlook.

Co-creation with patients allows the design of the artificial womb to go beyond medical and technical specifications to address the emotional and psychological needs of families. Parents will prioritize features that support bonding, such as ways to see and interact with their baby during development in the artificial womb. Additionally, they will emphasize safety, wanting assurances that the system provides the best possible care for their child while minimizing risks.

By engaging parents in the design process, the development of the artificial womb becomes more patient-centered, which can lead to greater acceptance and trust in the technology. This collaborative approach ensures that the final product not only functions effectively from a medical standpoint but also aligns with the desires and concerns of those who will ultimately use it, facilitating a smoother and faster implementation in clinical settings.

10.9 Reducing the Cost of Prematurity

In addition to its ethical benefits, artificial womb technology offers substantial economic advantages. The cost savings associated with reducing the need for extensive nursing care and optimizing resource utilization are significant. Preterm birth currently imposes immense financial burdens on healthcare systems worldwide, with annual costs estimated in the billions of dollars. By lowering the overall costs of neonatal care, this technology makes high-quality care more accessible and sustainable. Healthcare systems can manage their resources more effectively, ensuring that even resource-limited settings can benefit from advanced medical technologies.

Preterm birth not only affects the immediate family but also places a considerable financial strain on society as a whole. The high costs of neonatal intensive care, prolonged hospital stays, and the need for specialized medical equipment contribute to the overall economic burden. Artificial womb technology aims to address these issues by providing a more efficient and effective way to care for premature infants. This technology can potentially reduce the length of hospital stays and the need for costly medical interventions, leading to significant cost savings for healthcare providers and insurers.

The economic impact of prematurity is staggering. Currently, the annual global costs associated with the care of premature infants are estimated to be in the billions of dollars. These costs encompass not only immediate medical care but also long-term healthcare expenses, special education needs, and lost economic productivity due to developmental delays and health complications. The long-term financial implications include ongoing medical treatments, therapies, and support services that preterm infants often require as they grow older. Additionally, families of premature infants may face lost income due to the need for one parent to stay home and provide care, further exacerbating the economic strain. The long-term financial implications include ongoing medical treatments, therapies, and support services that preterm infants often require as they grow older. However, with the artificial womb's potential to improve neonatal outcomes, there may also be significant cost savings in the prevention of chronic diseases, such as hypertension and diabetes mellitus, which are commonly associated with low birth weight and can lead to substantial healthcare expenditures later in life.

Artificial womb technology offers a promising solution to these economic challenges. By improving the survival rates and health outcomes of premature infants, this technology can significantly reduce the long-term costs associated with prematurity. The advanced monitoring and support systems within the artificial womb create an optimal environment for fetal development, reducing the incidence of complications that typically arise from preterm birth. This not only improves the immediate health of the infant but also mitigates the need for long-term medical interventions and support.

The savings achieved through the adoption of artificial wombs can be redirected toward other critical healthcare needs, further enhancing the overall efficiency and sustainability of healthcare systems. This reallocation of resources can lead to improvements in other areas of maternal and child health, allowing for broader implementation of preventative care and early intervention programs. Additionally, the reduction in healthcare costs associated with prematurity can free up funds for research and development of new medical technologies, fostering innovation and advancement in the field of neonatal care.

The implementation of artificial womb technology not only has the potential to save countless lives but also to alleviate the economic burden on healthcare systems globally. By making high-quality neonatal care more accessible and affordable, this innovative technology paves the way for a future where the costs of premature birth are no longer an overwhelming financial burden. The benefits extend beyond immediate cost savings, offering a more sustainable and efficient approach to healthcare that can improve outcomes for premature infants and their families while strengthening healthcare systems worldwide.

10.10   Setting New Benchmarks in Healthcare

The artificial womb represents a paradigm shift in how healthcare challenges are addressed. It sets a new benchmark for medical research and clinical practice by harnessing the latest advancements in physiological and mathematical modeling, as well as artificial intelligence. This integrated approach ensures that medical procedures are not only safe and effective but also efficient and scalable. The vision for artificial womb technology is comprehensive and ambitious. It envisions a future where all incubators are eventually replaced by artificial wombs, providing an environment that supports the fetus' development until full maturity. This approach not only addresses the immediate needs of extremely premature infants but also offers a solution for late preterm infants, who often face developmental challenges. By fostering better developmental outcomes and improving bonding opportunities with parents, artificial wombs can give every child a stronger start in life.

10.11   A Brighter and Healthier Future

In summary, the advancement of artificial womb technology represents a significant step forward in medical science. It provides a precise, ethical, and efficient solution for neonatal care, with the potential to save many lives and improve healthcare practices globally. This innovation addresses current challenges and sets a new standard for future medical research and clinical applications. The artificial womb is not just a technological achievement; it is a crucial development that promises a better future for neonatal care.

One of the key benefits of this development is the reduction in the use of animal experiments. By utilizing advanced simulations and digital twin methodologies, medical teams can implement innovations more safely and effectively. These simulations allow researchers and clinicians to test and refine new technologies in a controlled, risk-free environment before applying them to patients. This approach can significantly enhance the implementation of medical advancements. Currently, it takes an average of 17 years for a medical innovation to be widely adopted, primarily due to the unfamiliarity of medical professionals with new technologies.

With the ability to practice extensively, as is now possible with the artificial womb, medical teams can become more comfortable and confident in using new technologies. This familiarity can lead to quicker adoption and integration of innovations into clinical practice, ultimately improving patient care. The artificial womb serves as a model for how other medical innovations can be safely developed and implemented. By practicing with these advanced systems, healthcare professionals can gain the necessary experience and trust to implement new applications more rapidly and safely in the clinical setting.

Moreover, the artificial womb's development showcases the potential for other areas of healthcare to benefit from similar advancements. For example, using simulation technology in surgery, drug development, and chronic disease management could drastically reduce the time it takes for these innovations to reach patients. The successful implementation of the artificial womb could thus pave the way for a new era in healthcare, where innovations are adopted more swiftly, benefiting patients and healthcare systems alike.

The economic benefits of this approach are also significant. By reducing the reliance on costly animal testing and streamlining the development and implementation of new technologies, healthcare systems can save substantial amounts of money. These savings can be redirected toward other critical areas of need, such as improving access to care, funding further research, and enhancing overall healthcare quality. The financial savings gained by reducing the need for intensive nursing care and improving resource efficiency are significant, helping to make high-quality care more widely available and sustainable.

The integration of artificial womb technology into neonatal care and medical research highlights a future focused on ethical considerations, resource efficiency, and improved health outcomes. This approach ensures that technological advancements provide the highest standard of care for the most vulnerable patients, giving every child the opportunity to thrive. The journey toward realizing this future underscores the importance of innovation and the ongoing commitment to enhancing human health and well-being across the healthcare sector.

In conclusion, the development and implementation of artificial womb technology mark a transformative leap in medical science, addressing the critical challenges of extreme preterm birth. This process, however, should always begin and end with the patient's needs. The journey starts with a question from the patient—how can we ensure the best possible outcome for premature infants?—and ends with an answer that meets both their emotional and medical expectations. Co-creation with patients is essential in this process. By involving parents in the design, safety, and bonding aspects of the artificial womb, we ensure that the technology aligns with their unique experiences and priorities. This patient-centered approach will not only create a product that better serves its users but also accelerate its acceptance and integration into clinical practice. By prioritizing the patient's voice throughout the innovation process, we reduce the time it takes for new technologies to be adopted, ensuring safe and effective implementation. Ultimately, co-creation fosters trust and support from those who will benefit most, paving the way for a smoother, faster, and more impactful revolution in neonatal care.

Appendix: A Comprehensive Guide to First-in-Human Trials of the Artificial Placenta Artificial Womb (APAW) Technology

Introduction

Extremely preterm birth, defined as birth before 28 weeks of gestation, remains one of the most significant challenges in neonatal care. Despite advances in neonatal intensive care unit (NICU) technology, outcomes for these infants often remain poor, with high rates of mortality and long-term morbidity. Underdeveloped lungs, fragile blood vessels, and immature organ systems make survival precarious, leaving many survivors with lifelong complications.

The artificial placenta artificial womb (APAW) system introduces a potentially transformative technology aimed at improving survival and long-term health outcomes for extremely preterm infants. By replicating the protective and nurturing environment of the uterus, the APAW system has the potential to bridge the gap between extreme prematurity and viability. This protocol outlines the structured, stepwise approach required to evaluate the safety, efficacy, and implementation of this novel technology.

1. *Preclinical validation*: Conduct extensive testing in animal models to refine the APAW system.
2. *Simulated trials*: Use high-fidelity mannequins and digital twin technology to simulate APAW usage in clinical scenarios.
3. *Regulatory approval*: Secure oversight from independent review boards and regulatory agencies.

G. Oei, *The Artificial Womb*, Copernicus Books, https://doi.org/10.1007/978-3-031-85905-2

4. *Training programs*: Develop comprehensive training for multidisciplinary medical teams.
5. *Pilot study*: Conduct a small-scale trial with strict monitoring to gather initial safety and efficacy data.
6. *Efficacy trials Randomized Controlled Trial (RCTs)*: Test the system's effectiveness in randomized controlled trials to provide robust evidence.
7. *Implementation study (Cohort Intervention Random Sampling Study [CIRSS])*: Use a cohort intervention random sampling study to evaluate real-world application and optimize widespread adoption.

Pilot Study Protocol

Objectives

- *Primary objective*: Assess initial safety of the APAW system over 28 days postdelivery in extremely preterm infants.
- *Secondary objectives*: Evaluate technical feasibility, parental satisfaction, and short-term outcomes.

Study Design

- Single-center, prospective pilot study.
- *Inclusion*: Infants born at 23 0/7 to 24 0/7 weeks of gestation.
- *Sample size*: Ten infants.
- *Intervention*: Transition into APAW within 30 minutes of birth, monitored for 28 days.
- *Outcome measures*: Survival without severe morbidity, infection rates, and system performance metrics.

Efficacy Trial (RCT) Protocol

Objectives

- *Primary objective*: Evaluate survival without severe neurodevelopmental impairment at 24 months corrected age.
- *Secondary objectives*: Assess growth parameters, respiratory outcomes, and NICU length of stay.

Study Design

- Multicenter, double-blind randomized controlled trial.
- *Inclusion*: Infants born at 23–26 weeks gestation.
- *Sample size*: 120 infants (60 APAW, 60 standard care).
- *Intervention*: APAW system usage for 28 days or until 28 weeks Postmenstrual Age (PMA).
- *Outcome measures*: Neurodevelopmental scores, incidence of complications (e.g., Intraventricular Hemorrhage (IVH), Necrotizing Enterocolitis (NEC)), and parental bonding metrics.

Sample Size

- Based on anticipated improvement in survival without severe morbidity from 25% in the standard NICU care group to 60% in the APAW group, with a two-sided alpha of 0.05 and 80% power:
  - 53 infants per group are required.
  - Accounting for a 10% dropout rate, the total sample size will be 120 infants (60 per group).

Implementation Study Protocol

Objectives

- *Primary objective*: Assess the effectiveness and scalability of APAW technology in routine clinical practice.
- *Secondary objectives*: Evaluate cost-effectiveness, accessibility, and integration into healthcare systems.

Study Design

- Cohort intervention random sampling study (CIRSS).
- *Intervention*: APAW system is provided to all eligible patients except a 10% randomly selected control group receiving standard NICU care.
- *Comparison*: Prospective APAW cohort versus retrospective standard care cohort.

- *Sample size*: 500 infants (450 APAW, 50 control).
- *Outcome measures*: Long-term health outcomes, patient demographics, and system scalability.

Rationale for CIRSS Design

CIRSS is chosen for the implementation phase due to its ability to

- Minimize bias by including nearly all eligible patients, compared to RCTs where only 5–10% of eligible participants typically enroll.
- Provide a real-world assessment of APAW performance, ensuring that findings are broadly applicable and not limited to a highly selective population.
- Use a small concurrent control group (10%) to confirm comparability with the historical cohort, reducing confounding while ensuring ethical feasibility.

Sample size calculation for CIRSS based on the anticipated improvement in survival without severe morbidity from 25% (historical cohort) to 60% (APAW group):

- *APAW group*: 450 infants.
- *Concurrent control group*: 50 infants (10% of the prospective cohort).
- *Historical control cohort*: Minimum of 500 infants from prior NICU care records.
- This design ensures sufficient statistical power to detect meaningful differences while addressing potential biases through causal inference methods and propensity score weighting.

Conclusion

This structured, stepwise approach ensures that the APAW system is rigorously evaluated, from initial safety assessments to real-world implementation. The pilot study will establish foundational data, efficacy trials will validate clinical benefits, and CIRSS implementation will ensure broad accessibility and integration. Together, these efforts aim to revolutionize neonatal care and offer new hope to families facing the challenges of extreme prematurity.

Contextual Note: An Illustrative Protocol

These clinical trial protocols serve as illustrative examples of how first-in-human studies for APAW technology might be designed. It provides a framework for researchers and clinicians considering similar trials, while also demonstrating the rigorous planning required for such innovative interventions. The methodology, sample size calculation, and ethical considerations outlined here are meant to inspire and guide further development rather than serve as a definitive, one-size-fits-all blueprint.

References

1. Adamson SL. Regulation of breathing at birth. J Dev Physiol. 1991;15:45–52.
2. American Bureau of shipping. Guidance Notes on Failure Mode and Effects Analysis (FMEA) for classification. 2015.
3. Amadei G, Handford CE, Qiu C, et al. Embryo model completes gastrulation to neurulation and organogenesis. Nature. 2022;610:143–53.
4. Arens J, Schnoering H, Pfennig M, et al. The Aachen MiniHLM—a miniaturized heart-lung machine for neonates with an integrated rotary blood pump. Artif Organs. 2010;34:707–13.
5. Arens J, Schoberer M, Lohr A, et al. NeonatOx—a pumpless extracorporeal lung support for premature neonates. Artif Organs. 2011;34:A8.
6. Armentrout D. Not ready for prime time: transitional events in the extremely preterm infant. J Perinat Neonatal Nurs. 2014;28:1449.
7. Awad JA, Cloutier R, Fournier L. Pumpless respiratory assistance using a membrane oxygenator as an artificial placenta: a preliminary study in newborn and preterm lambs. J Investig Surg. 1995;8:21–30.
8. Bartlett RH, Roloff DW, Cornell RG, Andrews PW, Dillon JB, Zwischenberger JB. Extracorporeal circulation in neonatal respiratory failure: a prospective randomized study. Pediatrics. 1985;76:479–87.
9. Bauer MS, Kirchner J. Implementation science: what is it and why should I care? Psychiatry Res. 2020;283:112376.
10. Blencowe H, Cousens S, Chou D, et al. Born too soon: the global epidemiology of 15 million preterm births. Reprod Health. 2013;10
11. Blencowe H, Cousens S, Oestergaard MZ, et al. National, regional, and worldwide estimates of preterm birth rates in the year 2010 with time trends since 1990 for selected countries: a systematic analysis and implications. Lancet. 2012;379:2162–72.

G. Oei, *The Artificial Womb*, Copernicus Books,
https://doi.org/10.1007/978-3-031-85905-2

12. Bioethics Journal. The ethics of ectogenesis. Bioethics J. 2020;34:328–30.
13. Callaghan JC, Angeles JD. Long-term extracorporeal circulation in the development of an artificial placenta for respiratory distress of the newborn. Surg Forum. 1961;12:215–7.
14. Callaghan JC, Cardozo D, Boracchia B, et al. Study of prepulmonary bypass in the development of an artificial placenta for prematurity and respiratory distress syndrome of the newborn. J Thorac Cardiovasc Surg. 1962;44:600–7.
15. Cannavò L, Rulli I, Falsaperla R, et al. Ventilation, oxidative stress and risk of brain injury in preterm newborns. Ital J Pediatr. 2020;46
16. Chalmers I, Enkin M, Keirse MJNC. Effective care in pregnancy and childbirth. Oxford University Press; 1989.
17. Charest-Pekeski AJ, Cho SKS, Aujla T, et al. Impact of the addition of a centrifugal pump in a preterm miniature pig model of the artificial placenta. Front Physiol. 2022;13
18. Colgrove N. Artificial womb technology and reproductive ethics. J Med Ethics. 2019;45:723–6.
19. Couzin-Frenkel J. Fluid-filled 'biobag' allows premature lambs to develop outside the womb: doctors looking ahead to human testing. Science. 2017; https://doi.org/10.1126/science.aal1101.
20. Crowther, C. Intrauterine blood transfusion for the treatment of red-cell isoimmunisation. Cochrane Database. 2004.
21. Dekker J, van Kaam AH, Roehr CC, et al. Stimulating and maintaining spontaneous breathing during transition of preterm infants. Pediatr Res. 2019:1–9.
22. De Bie FR, Davey MG, Larson AC, et al. Artificial placenta and womb technology: past, current, and future challenges towards clinical translation. Prenat Diagn. 2021;41:145–58.
23. De Bie FR, Kim SD, Bose SK, et al. Ethical considerations regarding artificial womb technology for the fetonate. Am J Bioeth. 2023;23(5):67–78.
24. Delnord M, Blondel B, Drewniak N, et al. Varying gestational age patterns in cesarean delivery: an international comparison. BMC Pregnancy Childbirth. 2014;14
25. Dominguez-Bello MG, De Jesus-Laboy KM, Shen N, et al. Partial restoration of the microbiota of cesarean-born infants via vaginal microbial transfer. Nat Med. 2016;22:250–3.
26. Dunn AB, Jordan S, Baker BJ, Carlson NS. The maternal-infant microbiome: considerations for labor and birth. MCN: American J Maternal/Child Nursing. 2017;42:318–25.
27. Eixarch E, Illa M, Fucho R, et al. An artificial placenta experimental system in sheep: critical issues for successful transition and survival up to one week. Biomedicines. 2023;11:702.
28. Elahi B. Safety risk management for medical devices. Elsevier; 2022.
29. Environmental science and technology. Sustainability of medical innovations. Environ J.

30. Finnemore A, Groves A. Physiology of the fetal and transitional circulation. Semin Fetal Neonatal Med. 2015;20:2106.

31. Fransen AF, van de Ven J, Schuit E, et al. Simulation-based team training for multi-professional obstetric care teams to improve patient outcomes: a multicentre, cluster randomized controlled trial. BJOG. 2016;124:641–50.

32. Gawande AA, Zinner MJ, Studdert DM, Brennan TA. Analysis of errors reported by surgeons at three teaching hospitals. Surgery. 2003;133:614–21.

33. Greenberg E. Patent granted in 1955 For the artificial uterus. Free patents.

34. Hooper SB, Te Pas AB, Kitchen MJ. Respiratory transition in the newborn: a three-phase process. Arch Dis Child Fetal Neonatal Ed. 2016;101:F266–71.

35. Jobe AH, Hillman N, Polglase G, Kramer BW, Kallapur S, Pillow J. Injury and inflammation from resuscitation of the preterm infant. Neonatology. 2008;94:190–6.

36. Kukora SK, Mychaliska GB, Weiss E M. Ethical challenges in first-in-human trials of the artificial placenta and artificial womb: not all technologies are created equally, ethically. J Perinatol. 2023.

37. Kuwabara Y, Okai T, Imanishi Y, Muronosono E, Kozuma S, Takeda S, Baba K, Mizuno M. Development of extrauterine fetal incubation system using extracorporeal membrane oxygenator. Artif Organs. 1987;11:224–7.

38. Lewis J, Schuh M, Hanna JH, Zernicka-Goetz M, Srivastava M, Tan T, Behjati S, et al. Developmental and stem cell biology's bright future. Cell. 2024;187:3224–8.

39. Liley AW. Intrauterine transfusion of the fetus in haemolytic disease. Br Med J. 1963;2:1107.

40. Liley, AW. The fetus as a personality. Eighth annual congress of the Australian and New Zealand college of psychiatry. 1971.

41. Mahony F, Hofmeyr GJ, Menon V. Choice of instruments for assisted vaginal delivery. Cochrane Database Syst Rev. 2010.

42. Matte GS, Connor KR, Toutenel NA, Gottlieb D, Fynn-Thompson FA. A modified EXIT-to-ECMO with optional reservoir circuit for use during an EXIT procedure requiring thoracic surgery. J Extracorporeal Technol. 2016;48:35–8.

43. Misra KB. Handbook of performability engineering. London: Springer; 2008.

44. Morton SU, Brodsky D. Fetal physiology and the transition to extrauterine life. Clin Perinatol. 2016;43:395–407.

45. Naeye RL. Umbilical cord length: clinical significance. J Pediatr. 1985;107:278–81.

46. Norman, DA. The Design of Everyday Things. Revised ed. Basic Books. 2013.

47. O'Brien SM, Mouser A, Odon JE, Winter C, Draycott TJ, Sumitro T, et al. Design and development of the BD Odon device™: a human factors evaluation process. BJOG. 2017;124:35–43.

48. Oldak B, Wildschutz E, Bondarenko V, Comar MY, Zhao C, Aguilera-Castrejon A, Tarazi S, Viukov S, et al. Complete human day 14 post-implantation embryo models from naive ES cells. Nature. 2023;622:562–73.

49. Partridge EA, et al. An extra-uterine system to physiologically support the extreme premature lamb. Nat Commun. 2017;8:15112.
50. Patel RM. Short- and long-term outcomes for extremely preterm infants. Am J Perinatol. 2016;33:318–28.
51. Reoma JL, Rojas A, Kim AC, et al. Development of an artificial placenta I: Pumpless arterio-venous extracorporeal life support in a neonatal sheep model. J Pediatr Surg. 2009;44:53–9.
52. Romanis EC. Artificial womb technology and the frontiers of human reproduction: conceptual differences and potential implications. J Med Ethics. 2018;44:751–5.
53. Romanis EC. Artificial womb technology and the choice to gestate ex utero: is partial ectogenesis the business of the criminal law? Med Law Rev. 2020;28:342–74.
54. Romanis EC. Artificial womb technology: conceptual and legal implications. J Law Biosci. 2021:8.
55. Sakata M, Hisano K, Okada M, Yasufuku M. A new artificial placenta with a centrifugal pump: long-term total extrauterine support of goat fetuses. J Thorac Cardiovasc Surg. 1998;115:1023–31.
56. Stricker BH. De geboorte van Horus, vol. I–V. Leiden: E.J. Brill; 1963–1989.
57. Tan CMJ, Lewandowski AJ. The transitional heart: from early embryonic and fetal development to neonatal life. Fetal Diagn Ther. 2020;47:373–86.
58. te Pas AB, Davis PG, Hooper SB, Morley CJ. From liquid to air: breathing after birth. J Pediatr. 2008;152:607–11.
59. Usuda H, et al. Successful maintenance of key physiological parameters in preterm lambs treated with ex vivo uterine environment therapy for a period of one week. Am J Obstet Gynecol. 2017;217:457.e1–457.e13.
60. van der Hout-van der Jagt MB, Verweij EJT, Andriessen P, de Boode WP, Bos AF, Delbressine FLM, et al. Interprofessional consensus regarding design requirements for liquid-based perinatal life support (PLS) technology. Front Pediatr. 2022;9.
61. van Haren JS, Delbressine FLM, Schoberer M, Te Pas AB, van Laar JOEH, Oei SG, et al. Transferring an extremely premature infant to an extra-uterine life support system: a prospective view on the obstetric procedure. Front Pediatr. 2024;12:1360111.
62. van Haren JS, van der Hout-van der Jagt MB, Meijer N, Monincx M, Delbressine FLM, Griffith XLG, et al. Simulation-based development: shaping clinical procedures for extra-uterine life support technology. Adv Simul. 2023;8:29.
63. van Willigen BG, van der Hout-van der Jagt MB, Huberts W, van de Vosse FN. A review study of fetal circulatory models to develop a digital twin of a fetus in a perinatal life support system. Front Pediatr. 2022;10.
64. Verrips M, van Haren JS, Oei SG, Moser A, van der Hout-van der Jagt MB. Clinical aspects of umbilical cord cannulation during transfer from the uterus to a liquid-based perinatal life support system for extremely premature infants: a qualitative generic study. PLoS One. 2023;18:e0290659.

65. Weizmann Institute of Science. Jacob Hanna's research on ectogenesis. Weizmann Institute Website.

66. Whalen M, Chang-Davidson E, Moran T, Hoffman R, Frydman GH, Slocum A, et al. Device prototype for vaginal delivery of extremely preterm fetuses in the breech presentation. J Med Devices. 2021;15

67. World Health Organization. Accessibility and equity in advanced reproductive technologies. WHO Report.

68. Zapol WM, Kolobow T, Pierce JG, Vurek GG, Bowman RL. Artificial placenta: two days of total extrauterine support of the isolated premature lamb fetus. Science. 1969;166:617–8.